CW00520255

The sirtfood diet

Cookbook

Complete guide to burn fat activating your 'skinny gene'. Tasty and healthy recipes to stay fit !

By Vilma J. Hernandez

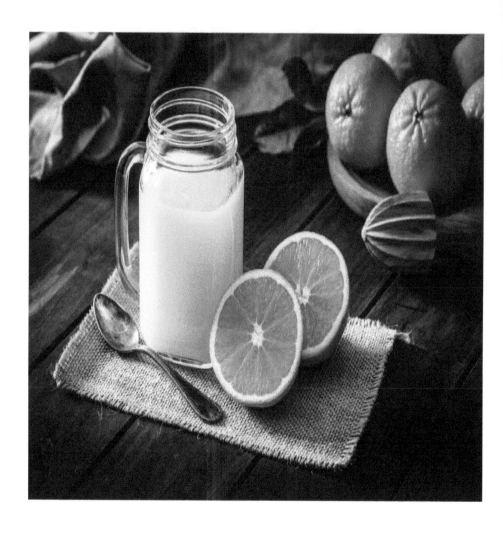

Introduction

The basis of the sirtuin diet can be explained in simple terms or complex ways. It is essential to understand how and why it works, however, to appreciate the value of what you are doing. It is also necessary to know why these sirtuin rich foods help you maintain fidelity to your diet plan. Otherwise, you may throw something in your meal with less nutrition that would defeat the purpose of planning for one rich in sirtuins. Most importantly, this is not a dietary fad, and as you will see, there is much wisdom in how humans have used natural foods even for medicinal purposes, over thousands of years.

To understand how the Sirtfood diet works and why these particular foods are necessary, we will look at their role in the human body.

Sirtuin activity was first researched in yeast, where a mutation caused an extension in the yeast's lifespan. Sirtuins were also shown to slow aging in laboratory mice, fruit flies, and nematodes. As Sirtuins' research proved to transfer to mammals, they were examined for their use in diet and slowing the aging process. The sirtuins in humans are different in typing, but they essentially work in the same ways and reasons.

There are seven "members" that make up the sirtuin family. It is believed that sirtuins play a significant role in regulating certain functions of cells, including proliferation (reproduction and growth of cells), apoptosis (death of cells). They promote survival and resist stress to increase longevity.

They are also seen to block neurodegeneration (loss of function of the brain's nerve cells). They conduct their housekeeping functions by cleaning out toxic proteins and supporting the brain's ability to change and adapt to different conditions or recuperate (i.e., brain plasticity). As part of this, they also help reduce chronic inflammation and reduce something called oxidative stress. Oxidative stress is when there are too many cell-damaging free radicals circulating in the body, and the body cannot catch up by combating them with anti-oxidants. These factors are related to age-related illness and weight, which again brings us back to how they work.

You will see labels in Sirtuins that start with "SIR," representing "Silence Information Regulator" genes. They do precisely that, silence or regulate, as part of their functions. The seven sirtuins humans work with are SIRT1, SIRT2, SIRT3, SIRT4, SIRT 5, SIRT6, and SIRT7. Each of these types is responsible for different areas of protecting cells. They work by either stimulating or turning on certain gene expressions or reducing and turning off other gene expressions. It essentially means that they can influence genes to do more or less of something, most of which they are already programmed to do.

Through enzyme reactions, each of the SIRT types affects different cells responsible for the metabolic processes that help maintain life. It is also related to what organs and functions they will act.

For example, SIRT6 causes the expression of the genes in humans that affect skeletal muscle, fat tissue, brain, and heart. SIRT 3 would induce an expression of genes that affect the kidneys, liver, brain, and heart.

If we tie these concepts together, you can see that the Sirtuin proteins can change the expression of genes, and in the case of the Sirtfood Diet, we care about how sirtuins can turn off those genes that are responsible for speeding up aging and for weight management.

The other aspect to this conversation of sirtuins is the function and the power of calorie restriction on the human body. Calorie restriction is merely eating fewer calories. It, coupled with exercise and reducing stress, is usually a combination of weight loss. Calorie restriction has also proven across much research in animals and humans to increase one's lifespan.

We can look further at the role of sirtuins with calorie restriction and using the SIRT3 protein, which has a role in metabolism and aging. Amongst all of the effects of the protein on gene expression (such as preventing cells from dying, reducing tumors from growing, etc.), we want to understand the impact of SIRT3 on weight for this book.

As we stated earlier, the SIRT3 has high expression in those metabolically active tissues, and its ability to express itself increases with caloric restriction, fasting, and exercise. On the contrary, it will express itself less when the body has high fat, high-calorie-riddled diet.

The last few highlights of sirtuins are their role in regulating telomeres and reducing inflammation, which also helps prevent disease and aging.

Telomeres are sequences of proteins at the ends of chromosomes. When cells divide, these get shorter. As we age, they get shorter, and other stressors to the body also will contribute to this. Maintaining these longer telomeres is the key to slower aging. Also, proper diet, along with exercise and other variables, can lengthen telomeres. SIRT6 is one of the sirtuins that, if activated, can help with DNA damage, inflammation, and oxidative stress. SIRT1 also helps with inflammatory response cycles that are related to many age-related diseases.

Calories restriction, as we mentioned earlier, can extend life to some degree. Since this and fasting are a stressor, these factors will stimulate the SIRT3 proteins to kick in and protect the body from the stressors and excess free radicals. Again, the telomere length is affected as well.

To sum up, all of this information also shows that, contrary to some people's beliefs, genetics, such as "it is what it is" or "it is my fate because Uncle Joe has something..." through our own lifestyle choices. To what we are exposed to, we can influence action and changes in our genes. It is quite an empowering thought, yet another reason you should be excited to have a science-based diet such as the Sirtfood diet is available to you.

Having laid this all out before you, you should be able to appreciate how and why these miraculous compounds work in your favor to keep you youthful, healthy, and lean. If they are working hard for you, don't you feel that you should do something too? Well, you can, and that is what the rest of this book will do for you by providing all the SIRT-recipes.

Chapter 1. The Advantages Of The Sirt Diet

Sirtuins are a group of 7 proteins that maintain cell metabolism and homeostasis at optimal levels. Three of these proteins are found in the mitochondria, the cytoplasm, and another three are located in the nucleus. Sirtuins maintain the cell's health and ensure that all processes going on within the cell are properly happening. Sirtuins can, however, not be effective without the presence of NAD+ (nicotinamide adenine dinucleotide). NAD+ is a coenzyme that is present in all cells that are living in nature. NAD+ ensures that Sirtuins function optimally and can regulate cells.

Homeostasis within the cell maintains all the numerous functions of the cell at stability, which ensures balance. It may also involve the maintenance of PH and the saturate concentration levels of the cytoplasm, which is the most significant cell component in terms of volume. All these are aspects of the cell that must stay constant for optimal cell health. Sirtuins perform several functions, among them being the ability to deacetylase proteins called histones. Acetyls are proteins with a physical form of Histones are proteins that contain a condensed form of DNA called chromatins, which prevent the proteins from performing their functions in this acetyl.

The deacetylation frees the proteins for their respective functions, given that proteins are the building blocks for the body. Proteins are proverbially referred to as bodybuilding foods. Without Sirtuins, therefore, the bodybuilding foods would fail to build our bodies as they are the critical components for freeing the protein molecules in our cells for their functions.

The Miracle of the Blue Areas

The other evidence for the power of Sirtfoods comes from the 'blue zones.' The blue zones are small regions in the world where people miraculously live longer than everywhere else.

Perhaps most startlingly, you don't just see people live longer in blue zones; you still see them retain energy, vigor, and overall health even in their advanced years. Many of us have a fear of becoming decrepit, immobile, and overall miserable as we age.

Furthermore, we envision this as starting to occur in our forties and fifties while becoming a fixed reality in our sixties, seventies, and eighties. Yet in the blue zones, people live past 100 surprisingly regularly but can walk, work and exercise just as well as those in the younger years. Likewise, they remain mentally capable and don't suffer the cognitive deficits we typically associate with old age.

The blue zones include several areas of the Mediterranean, Japan, Italy, and Costa Rica. What do these regions all have in common? They all eat a diet high in Sirt foods. The Mediterranean is famous for its healthy diet involving copious amounts of fish and olive oil. The Japanese savor matcha green tea, while the Costa Ricans traditionally indulge in cocoa, coffee, and more.

The beauty of the Sirt food diet isn't trying to make your eating habits artificial and awkward. It is merely copying the healthiest practices that already exist around the world.

Sirt Diet and Muscle Mass

There is a family of genes that function as guardians of our muscle in the body. Also, when under stress, avoid its breakdown, it is known as the sirtuins. SIRT is a potent Muscle Breakdown Inhibitor. As long as SIRT is activated, even when we are fasting, muscle breakdown is prevented, and we continue to burn fat for fuel.

SIRT's benefits aren't ending with preserving muscle mass. The sirtuins work to increase our skeletal muscle mass. We need to explore into the exciting world of stem cells and illustrate how that process functions. Our muscle comprises a particular type of stem cell called a satellite cell that regulates its development and regeneration. Satellite cells sit there quietly most of the time, but they are activated when a muscle gets damaged or stressed. By things like weight training, this is how our muscles grow stronger. SIRT is essential for activating satellite cells, and without its activity, muscles are significantly smaller because they no longer have the capacity to develop or regenerate properly. However, by increasing SIRT activity, we boost our satellite cells, encouraging muscle growth and recovery.

Sirt Diet and Goodness

There was one aspect we couldn't get our minds around in our pilot study: the people didn't get hungry given a drop-in calorie. In reality, several people struggled to consume all of the food that was offered.

One of the significant advantages of the Sirtfood Diet is that we can achieve significant benefits without the need for a long-term calorie restriction. The very first week of diet is the process of hyper-success, where we pair mild fasting with an excess of strong Sirtfoods for a double blow to weight. So, we predicted sure signs of hunger here, as with all of the fasting regimens. But we've had virtually zero!

We found the answer as we trawled through analysis. It's all thanks to the body's primary appetite-regulating hormone, leptin, called the "satiety hormone." As we feed, leptin decreases, signaling the hypothalamus inhibiting desire to a part of the brain. Conversely, leptin signaling to the mind declines as we fly, which makes us feel thirsty.

Leptin is so effective in controlling appetite that early expectations where it could be treated as a "magic bullet" for combating obesity. But that vision was broken because the metabolic disorder found in obesity causes leptin to avoid correctly functioning. Through obesity, the volume of leptin that can reach the brain is not only decreased. But the hypothalamus also becomes desensitized to its behavior. It is regarded as leptin resistance: there is leptin, but it doesn't work correctly anymore. Therefore, for many overweight individuals, the brain continues to think they are underfed even though they consume plenty, which triggers them to seek calories.

The consequence of this is that while the amount of leptin in the blood is necessary to control appetite, how much of it enters the brain and can affect the hypothalamus is far more relevant. It is here that the Sirtfoods shine.

New evidence indicates that the nutrients present in Sirtfoods have unique advantages in overcoming leptin resistance. By increasing leptin delivery to the brain and through the hypothalamus ' response to leptin behavior.

Going back to our original question on why don't the Sirtfood Diet make people feel hungry? Given a decrease in blood leptin rates during the mild quick, which would usually raise motivation, incorporating Sirtfoods into the diet makes leptin signals more productive, leading to better appetite control. Sirtfoods also have powerful effects on our taste centers, meaning we get a lot more pleasure and satisfaction from our food. Therefore, don't fall into the overeating trap to feel happy. Sirtuins are expected to be a brand-new concept for even the most committed dietitians. But hitting the sirtuins, our metabolism's master regulators, is the foundation of any effective diet for weight loss. Tragically, the very existence of our modern society, with abundant food and sedentary lifestyles, creates a perfect storm to shut down our sirtuin operation, and we see all around us the effects of this.

The good thing is that we know what sirtuins are, how fat accumulation is managed, and how fat burning is encouraged, and most significantly, how to turn them on. And with this revolutionary breakthrough, the key to successful and lasting weight loss is now yours to bear.

Maintaining The Sirtfood Diet

After the successful beginning of the Sirtfood diet, there is more work to do. You need to ensure that the morale and momentum you had at the beginning of the diet are maintained to complete the diet. In this regard, the tips given have been tested and confirmed to help people manage the motivation and morale for completing the Sirtfood diet.

Check-In with Your Set Goals

You have understood the importance of setting goals at the inception of the Sirtfood diet. These goals need to attainable and realistic to allow for adherence to it. However, these realistic goals that you have set need to be checked continuously during the diet. Continually checking in with your set goals reminds you of the reason for starting the diet in the first place. It brings up the image of the future you had in mind at the beginning of the Sirtfood diet. By checking your set target during the diet course, the primary source of motivation and inspiration for the diet is revived, thus giving you enough will continue with the Sirtfood diet no matter the difficulties encountered.

Apart from reviving the motivation for continuing the Sirtfood diet, reviewing your goals allows you to track your diet's progress. Remember that while drawing up your plans, the processes and pathways are also defined. These defined pathways are used to monitor your progress with the Sirtfood diet.

Understand That It Is Acceptable to Make Mistakes

One of the banes of most dieters is cheating or eating off-plan. It occurs when they eat foods that are not in tandem with the dictates of their diet. In the Sirtfood diet, it is possible to eat off-plan too. There are days you may overeat or eat wrongly due to forgetfulness, and some days you may give in to your cravings. If and when any of these occasions, do not be too hard on yourself and do not lose hope. It would help if you remembered that you are only human, and it is acceptable to make mistakes. Most importantly, you must remember that the most vital and helpful step you can take after eating out of the diet is to pick up yourself and learn from your mistakes.

You need to understand the reason for the relapse. Was it due to cravings or forgetfulness? What exactly went wrong? Getting answers to these questions will help you map out the steps that you must take to avoid such relapse afterward. For instance, if the mistake was due to forgetfulness, you can set up periodic reminders to always keep you in check at all times.

On the other hand, if the mistake was born out of cravings, you may need to talk to your dietician. The dietician will help you find out if the craving's food items can hurt the Sirtfood diet plans. It will help provide options and solutions to overcome this mistake.

In summary, after making a mistake with the diet plan, the next course of action should be how to overcome the error and prevent future occurrences.

Combine Exercises with The Sirtfood Diet

Exercises are very beneficial to human health. Combining it with a healthy diet like the Sirtfood diet increases the health benefits that can be derived. However, exercising regularly during the diet has immense health benefits and helps you stay focused on a diet. You may wonder how that works.

By combining exercise with the Sirtfood diet, there is a considerable likelihood of quickly and easily achieving your set goals. For people going into the Sirtfood diet to achieve healthy weight loss, exercising is a great plus that quickly achieves this goal. Also, exercises help you accomplish this accessible for people going into the diet for the energy-boosting effect.

When your set goals are achieved easily during the Sirtfood diet, the zeal to remain focused and maintain the diet is renewed. The possibility of getting discouraged during the dieting process is reduced as you can see the diet's achievements.

Smart Snacking

While on a diet such as the Sirtfood diet, there is a restriction on what to eat and drink. Hence, in situations where you need to be away from home for an extended period, you need to ensure that you have a reliable source of Sirtfoods to eat when the need arises. Because it is not very comfortable to pack food items with you wherever you go, snacks remain the best and most suitable option.

Snacks and fast food are handy in serving as an alternative to real foods when the need arises. However, not all snacks can be used in place of Sirtfoods. It is the origination of the concept of smart snacks.

Smart snacks are healthy and appropriate alternatives that can be used in place of Sirtfoods, especially when you are away from home or cannot access your Sirtfood items. Snacking is another way of maintaining the Sirtfood diet. By having smart snacks on you whenever you are far from home, you have the opportunity to feed your body with needed nutrients through the smart snack without eating unhealthy food or out of the Sirtfood diet.

Make the Best Out of Your Restaurant Time

Sometimes, it is impossible to have access to smart snacks. It may be due to forgetfulness on your part, or you cannot afford to get some because of time or space. In most cases, the only option you are left with at this point is to eat out or starve until you get home. Of course, starving yourself is not an ideal option as it undermines your strength to carry out your work and other activities effectively.

The viable choice here is to eat at a restaurant. As discouraging as it may sound to your Sirtfood diet plan, you can still attempt to make the best out of it. Make inquiries about the availability of some Sirtfoods in the restaurant. While some particular foods are peculiar to the Sirtfood diet, some general food items are also sirtuin-friendly. Try to get these foods if you can.

However, if these foods are not available, opt-in for nutritious or healthy foods; although these foods are not Sirtfoods, they are filled with essential nutrients that will do your body a whole lot of good. If these foods and fruits are available at your eat-out spot or restaurant, they are safe for you to eat.

If the restaurants do not have these types of food in stock, you can eat whatever pleases you on the menu. It is the other best option other than starving yourself. However, you remember that you need to balance this episode of eating out with sufficient Sirtfoods so that your goals are not affected.

Mind What You Eat

There is a practice called mindful eating. It involves people paying detailed and intricate attention to what they eat and its effect on their bodies. To some school of thought, mindful eating is a diet with some health benefits. While I will not precisely classify mindful eating as a diet type, there is no doubt that it has some advantages, health-wise. These benefits, among other things, will help you stay focused on your Sirtfood diet.

By practicing mindful eating, the body is put to receive more nutrients and less unhealthy elements. It is because mindful eating requires researching thoroughly into the nutritional constituents of what we eat. By doing so, nutritious and beneficial foods are distinguished from unhealthy food. Since it is unlikely that anyone would knowingly consume unhealthy foods, more nutrients are fed into the body by eating healthy foods.

Feeding the body with enough nutrients helps maintain the Sirtfood diet. With abundant nutrient in the body, the benefits of the diet can easily be achieved and sustained. Therefore, if you wish to maintain the Sirtfood diet, you can practice mindful eating to help with the process.

Stick to The Sirtfood Diet Plan

This point sounds like a no-brainer, but it is crucial and requires reiteration. Sticking to the diet plan is one sure way of ensuring that both short-term and long-term goals of the diet are achieved.

Sticking to the diet plan from the inception of the Sirtfood diet is instrumental in attaining the short-term goals. These goals include drastic but healthy weight loss and improvement in the body's energy level, among other things. Apart from their inherent health benefits, the attainment of these goals is a significant boost to anyone's morale under this diet. Seeing that some of the goals set at the beginning of the diet have been achieved, remaining focused and maintaining the diet would be less stressful. Hence sticking to the diet plan is a vital step in ensuring that you retain the Sirtfood diet.

Furthermore, the success of all the tips recently given is dependent on your ability to stick with the diet plan. Without the determination to stick to the diet plan, all the other suggestions will be useless and ineffective.

These tips given help you maintain the zeal and momentum for the Sirtfood diet. This way, the successful completion of the dieting process is ensured.

Vilma J. Hernandez © Copyright 2021 - All rights reserved.

The content contained within this book may not be reproduced, duplicated or transmitted without direct written permission from the author or the publisher.

Under no circumstances will any blame or legal responsibility be held against the publisher, or author, for any damages, reparation, or monetary loss due to the information contained within this book. Either directly or indirectly.

Legal Notice:

This book is copyright protected. This book is only for personal use. You cannot amend, distribute, sell, use, quote or paraphrase any part, or the content within this book, without the consent of the author or publisher.

Disclaimer Notice:

Please note the information contained within this document is for educational and entertainment purposes only. All effort has been executed to present accurate, up to date, and reliable, complete information. No warranties of any kind are declared or implied. Readers acknowledge that the author is not engaging in the rendering of legal, financial, medical or professional advice. The content within this book has been derived from various sources. Please consult a licensed professional before attempting any techniques outlined in this book.

By reading this document, the reader agrees that under no circumstances is the author responsible for any losses, direct or indirect, which are incurred as a result of the use of information contained within this document, including, but not limited to, — errors, omissions, or inaccuracies.

Table of Contents

INTRODUCTION 4

CHAPTER 1. THE ADVANTAGES OF THE SIRT DIET...................**15**

THE MIRACLE OF THE BLUE AREAS...18

SIRT DIET AND MUSCLE MASS...21

SIRT DIET AND GOODNESS...24

MAINTAINING THE SIRTFOOD DIET **31**

CHAPTER 1. SNACKS 56

1.   CELERY AND RAISINS SNACK SALAD.................................56

2.   DILL AND BELL PEPPERS SNACK BOWL 58

3.   SPICY PUMPKIN SEEDS BOWL 60

4.   APPLE AND PECAN BOWLS 61

5.   ZUCCHINI BOWLS...62

6.   CHEESY MUSHROOMS...64

7.   MOZZARELLA CAULIFLOWER BARS 66

8.   CINNAMON APPLE CHIPS 68

9.   VEGETABLE AND NUTS BREAD LOAF 69

10.   EASY CRACKERS 71

11.   ALMOND CRACKERS 73

12.   MONKEY TRAIL MIX 75

13.   GRANOLA WITH QUINOA...77

14. MED-STYLED OLIVES 79

15. ROASTED CHICKPEAS 81

16. BAKED ROOT VEG CRISPS 83

17. LEMON RICOTTA COOKIES WITH LEMON GLAZE 86

18. PEANUT BUTTER SNACK BALLS 89

19. MASCARPONE CHEESECAKE WITH ALMOND CRUST 91

20. PIZZA KALE CHIPS 94

21. TUSCAN BEAN STEW 97

22. CHOCOLATE NUT TRUFFLES 99

23. CHOCOLATE BALLS 101

24. VANILLA CRÈME BRULE 103

25. HEALTHY COFFEE COOKIES 106

26. STRAWBERRY OATMEAL BARS 109

27. PARSLEY CHEESE BALLS 112

28. BAKED KALE CHIPS 114

CHAPTER 2. SAUCES & DIPS 116

29. SWEET AND SAVORY CHERRY COMPOTE 116

30. CILANTRO LIME SAUCE 118

31. GREEK TZATZIKI SAUCE 120

32. GREEN ENCHILADA SAUCE 122

33. JALAPENO PINEAPPLE AIOLI 124

34.	AWESOME SAUCE	126
35.	VEGAN HOLLANDAISE SAUCE	128
36.	VEGAN CHEESE SAUCE	130
37.	TERIYAKI SAUCE	132
38.	THAI PEANUT SAUCE	134
39.	TASTY VEGAN GRAVY	136

CHAPTER 3. JUICES & SMOOTHIES 139

40.	KALE KIWI SMOOTHIE	139
41.	SALAD SMOOTHIE	141
42.	AVOCADO KALE SMOOTHIE	143
43.	KALE BANANA APPLE SMOOTHIE	145
44.	KALE CUCUMBER APPLE SMOOTHIE	147
45.	GRAPEFRUIT KALE SMOOTHIE	149
46.	PEAR CILANTRO SMOOTHIE	151
47.	KEFIR KALE BANANA ORANGE CHIA SMOOTHIE	153
48.	MATCHA APPLE & GREENS JUICE	155
49.	CELERY JUICE	157
50.	APPLE, CUCUMBER & CELERY JUICE	159
51.	LEMONY APPLE & KALE JUICE	160
52.	ORANGE JUICE	162
53.	APPLE & CUCUMBER JUICE	164
54.	APPLE & CELERY JUICE	165

55. APPLE, ORANGE & BROCCOLI JUICE 166

56. APPLE, GRAPEFRUIT & CARROT JUICE 167

57. GREEN FRUIT JUICE.. 169

58. APPLE & CARROT JUICE.. 171

59. LEMONY GREEN JUICE.. 172

60. SIRTFOOD SMOOTHIE... 174

61. STRAWBERRY JUICE 176

62. CHOCOLATE DATE SMOOTHIE..................................... 177

63. BLUEBERRY & KALE SMOOTHIE................................... 179

64. STRAWBERRY & BEET SMOOTHIE............................... 181

65. GREEN PINEAPPLE SMOOTHIE 183

66. MANGO SMOOTHIE.. 184

67. RED WINE HOT CHOCOLATE 185

68. CITRIC BLUEBERRY SLUSH... 187

69. CITRUS, BLUEBERRY & ROSEMARY MOCKTAIL......... 188

70. SPICED GREEN TEA TONIC... 190

71. GREEN TEA SMOOTHIE 192

72. MINT, LEMON, AND BLUEBERRY INFUSED WATER... 193

73. MINT-CITRUS ICED TEA... 195

74. CUCUMBER, LEMON KIWI AGUA FRESCA.................... 197

75. MINT, CUCUMBER, LIME, AND STRAWBERRY INFUSED
WATER.. 199

76. APPLE TEA.. 201

CHAPTER 5. DESSERTS **202**

77. BAKED POMEGRANATE CHEESECAKE 202

78. MERINGUES WITH BLACK CURRANTS 206

79. BLACK CURRANT AND RASPBERRY GRANITA 208

80. CHOCOLATE AND BLACKBERRY MINI PAVLOVAS 210

81. CHOCOLATE MOUSSE 213

82. GREEN ICED TEA ICE-CREAM 216

83. POMEGRANATE AND BLUEBERRY RICE 218

84. CHOCOLATE APPLE CAKE 219

85. BLUEBERRY FUN 221

86. BERRY GOOD! 223

87. SNOWFLAKES 225

88. HOME-MADE MARSHMALLOW FLUFF 226

89. BANANA ICE CREAM 229

90. DARK CHOCOLATE PRETZEL COOKIES 231

CONCLUSION **233**

Chapter 1. Snacks

1. Celery and Raisins Snack Salad

Preparation time: 15 minutes

Cooking time: 0 minutes

Servings: 4

Ingredients:

- ½ cup raisins

- 4 cups celery, sliced

- ¼ cup parsley, chopped

- ½ cup walnuts, chopped

- Juice of ½ lemon

- 2 tablespoons olive oil

- Salt and black pepper to the taste

Directions:

1. In a salad bowl, mix celery with raisins, walnuts, parsley, lemon juice, oil, and black pepper and toss. Divide into small cups and serve as a snack.

Nutrition:

Calories: 150

Carbs: 30g

Fat: 4g

Protein: 2g

2. Dill and Bell Peppers Snack Bowl

Preparation time: 15 minutes

Cooking time: 0 minutes

Servings: 4

Ingredients:

- 2 tablespoons dill, chopped

- 1 yellow onion, chopped

- 1-pound multi-colored bell peppers, cut into halves, seeded, and cut into thin strips

- 3 tablespoons extra virgin olive oil

- 2 and ½ tablespoons white vinegar

- Black pepper to the taste

Directions:

1. In a salad bowl, mix bell peppers with onion, dill, pepper, oil, vinegar, and toss to coat. Divide into small bowls and serve as a snack.

Nutrition:

Calories: 25

Carbs: 5g

Fat: 0g

Protein: 1g

3. Spicy Pumpkin Seeds Bowl

Preparation time: 5 minutes

Cooking time: 20 minutes

Servings: 6

Ingredients:

- ½ tablespoon chili powder

- ½ teaspoon cayenne pepper

- 2 cups pumpkin seeds

- 2 teaspoons lime juice

Directions:

1. Spread pumpkin seeds on a lined baking sheet, add lime juice, cayenne, chili powder, and toss well. Put it in the oven and roast at 275 degrees F for 20 minutes. Divide into small bowls and serve as a snack.

Nutrition:

Calories: 150

Carbs: 3g Fat: 13g .Protein: 8g

4. Apple and Pecan Bowls

Preparation time: 15 minutes

Cooking time: 0 minutes

Servings: 4

Ingredients:

- 4 big apples, cored, peeled, and cubed

- 2 teaspoons lemon juice

- ¼ cup pecans, chopped

Directions:

1. Mix apples with lemon juice and pecans in a bowl and toss. Divide into small bowls and serve as a snack.

Nutrition:

Calories: 78

Carbs: 13g

Fat: 2g

Protein: 1g

5. Zucchini Bowls

Preparation time: 15 minutes

Cooking time: 20 minutes

Servings: 12

Ingredients:

- Cooking spray

- ½ cup dill, chopped

- 1 egg

- ½ cup whole wheat flour

- Black pepper to the taste

- 1 yellow onion, chopped

- 2 garlic cloves, minced

- 3 zucchinis, grated

Directions:

1. In a bowl, mix zucchinis with garlic, onion, flour, pepper, egg, and dill and stir well. Shape the mix into

12 portions with small bowls' help and arrange them on a lined baking sheet.

2. Grease them with some cooking spray and bake at 400 degrees F for 20 minutes, flipping them halfway. Serve at room temperature as snacks.

Nutrition:

Calories: 108

Carbs: 15g

Fat: 3g

6. Cheesy Mushrooms

Preparation time: 15 minutes

Cooking time: 20 minutes

Servings: 5

Ingredients:

- 20 white mushroom caps

- 1 garlic clove, minced

- 3 tablespoons parsley, chopped

- 2 yellow onions, chopped

- Black pepper to the taste

- ½ cup low-fat parmesan, grated

- ¼ cup low-fat mozzarella, grated

- A drizzle of olive oil

- 2 tablespoons non-fat yogurt

Directions:

1. Heat-up a pan with some oil over medium heat, add garlic and onion, stir, cook for 10 minutes and transfer to a bowl.

2. Add black pepper, garlic, parsley, mozzarella, parmesan, and yogurt, stir well, stuff the mushroom caps with the mix.

3. Arrange them on a lined baking sheet and bake in the oven at 400 degrees F for 20 minutes. Serve.

Nutrition:

Calories: 181

Carbs: 1g

Fat: 16g

Protein: 9g

7. Mozzarella Cauliflower Bars

Preparation time: 15 minutes

Cooking time: 20 minutes

Servings: 12

Ingredients:

- 1 big cauliflower head, riced

- ½ cup low-fat mozzarella cheese, shredded

- ¼ cup egg whites

- 1 teaspoon Italian seasoning

- Black pepper to the taste

Directions:

1. Spread the riced cauliflower on a lined baking sheet and cook in the oven at 375 degrees F for 20 minutes.

2. Transfer to a bowl, add black pepper, cheese, seasoning, and egg whites, stir, spread into a rectangle pan, and press well on the bottom.

3. Introduce in the oven at 375 degrees F and bake for 20 minutes. Let it cool and slice into 12 bars. Serve at room temperature as a snack.

Nutrition:

Calories: 319

Carbs: 34g

Fat: 17g

Protein: 7g

8. Cinnamon Apple Chips

Preparation time: 15 minutes

Cooking time: 2 hours

Servings: 4

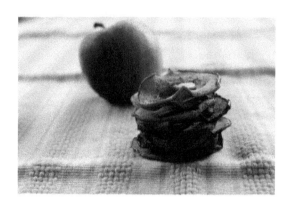

Ingredients:

- Cooking spray

- 2 teaspoons cinnamon powder

- 2 apples, cored and thinly sliced

Directions:

1. Arrange apple slices on a lined baking sheet, spray them with cooking oil, and sprinkle cinnamon on it. Put it in the oven and bake at 300 degrees F for 2 hours. Divide into bowls and serve as a snack.

Nutrition:

Calories: 140

Carbs: 20g

Fat: 7g

Protein: 0g

9. Vegetable and Nuts Bread Loaf

Preparation time: 15 minutes

Cooking time: 1 hour & 35 minutes

Servings: 4

Ingredients:

- 6oz mushrooms, finely chopped

- 3½ oz haricot beans

- 3½ oz walnuts, finely chopped

- 3½ oz peanuts, finely chopped

- 1 carrot, finely chopped

- 3 sticks celery, finely chopped

- 1 bird's-eye chili, finely chopped

- 1 red onion, finely chopped

- 1 egg, beaten

- 2 cloves of garlic, chopped

- 2 tablespoons olive oil

- 2 teaspoons turmeric powder

- 2 tablespoons soy sauce

- 4 tablespoons fresh parsley, chopped

- 100mls (3½ Fl oz) water

- 60mls (2fl oz) red wine

Directions:

1. Warm oil in a pan and add the garlic, chili, carrot, celery, onion, mushrooms, and turmeric. Cook for 5 minutes. Place the haricot beans in a bowl and stir in nuts, vegetables, soy sauce, egg, parsley, red wine, and water.

2. Grease and line a large loaf tin with greaseproof paper. Spoon the batter into the loaf tin, cover with foil and bake in the oven at 375F for 60-90 minutes. Let it stand within 10 minutes, then turn onto a serving plate.

Nutrition:

Calories: 83

Carbs: 16g Fat: 2g Protein: 2g

10. Easy Crackers

Preparation time: 15 minutes

Cooking time: 60 minutes

Servings: 72 crackers

Ingredients:

- 1 cup boiling water
- 1/3 cup chia seeds
- 1/3 cup sesame seeds
- 1/3 cup pumpkin seeds
- 1/3 cup Flaxseeds
- 1/3 cup sunflower seeds
- 1 tablespoon Psyllium powder
- 1 cup almond flour
- 1 teaspoon salt
- ¼ cup coconut oil, melted

Directions:

1. Preheat your oven to 300 degrees F.

2. Add listed fixing except coconut oil and water to the food processor and pulse until ground. Transfer to a mixing bowl, then pour melted coconut oil and boiling water, mix.

3. Transfer mix to prepared sheet and spread into a thin layer. Cut dough into crackers and bake for 60 minutes. Cool and serve as needed as a snack.

Nutrition:

Calories: 180

Carbs: 28g

Fat: 5g

Protein: 4g

11. Almond Crackers

Preparation time: 15 minutes

Cooking time: 20 minutes

Servings: 40 crackers

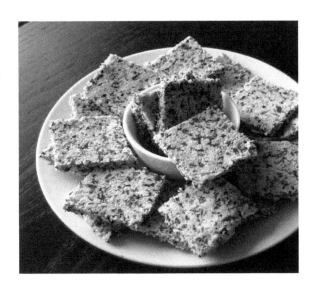

Ingredients:

- 1 cup almond flour

- ¼ teaspoon baking soda

- 1/8 teaspoon black pepper

- 3 tablespoons sesame seeds

- 1 egg, beaten

- Salt and pepper to taste

Directions:

1. Warm your oven to 350 degrees F. Line two baking sheets with parchment paper and keep them on the side.

2. Mix the dry ingredients in a large bowl and add egg, mix well and form a dough. Divide dough into two balls. Roll out the dough between two pieces of parchment paper.

3. Cut into crackers and transfer them to the prepared baking sheet. Bake for 15-20 minutes. Repeat until all the dough has been used up. Leave crackers to cool and serve as needed.

Nutrition:

Calories: 130

Carbs: 5g

Fat: 11g

Protein: 6g

12. Monkey Trail Mix

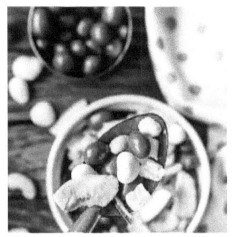

Preparation Time: 1 hour

Cooking Time: 30 minutes.

Servings: 5

Ingredients:

- 1 teaspoon of vanilla extract

- 3 tablespoons of coconut oil

- 1/3 cup of coconut sugar

- 6 oz. of dried banana

- ½ cup of dark chocolate chips

- 1 cup of coconut flakes, unsweetened

- 1 cup of cashews, raw and unsalted

- 2 cups of walnuts, raw and unsalted

Directions:

1. Add the coconut oil, vanilla extract, coconut sugar, coconut flakes, and nuts into a crockpot. Stir to combine, then cook on high for 1 hour. Stir occasionally to make sure the coconut flakes do not burn.

2. Turn the crockpot temperature to low and continue to cook for another 30 minutes. Put the batter out onto parchment paper and allow to dry completely.

3. Allow the mixture to cool before adding the banana and chocolate chips. Store in an airtight container and enjoy when hungry.

4. Use a combination of raw, unsalted nuts to extend the recipe — this can include Brazil nuts or almonds.

Nutrition:

Calories: 151

Fat: 10g

Carbs: 13g

Protein: 4g

13. Granola with Quinoa

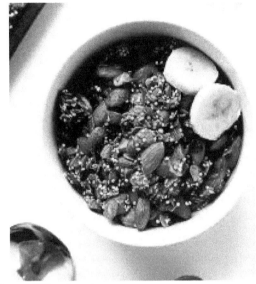

Preparation Time: 30 minutes

Cooking Time: 20 minutes

Servings: 6

- 1 pinch of salt

- ¼ cup of maple syrup

- 3 ½ tablespoons of coconut oil

- 1 tablespoon coconut sugar

- 1 cup of rolled oats

- 2 cups of almonds, raw and unsalted

- ½ cup of quinoa, uncooked

Directions:

1. Warm your oven to 340 F and line a baking tray with parchment paper. In a large mixing bowl, add the salt, sugar, oats, almonds, and quinoa and set aside.

2. In a small saucepan over medium heat, add the maple syrup and coconut oil. Using a whisk, stir until combined, then remove from the heat.

3. Pour the syrup over the mixed nuts and quinoa and give it a thorough stir. Place the mixture onto the baking tray and, using a spatula, spread the ingredients evenly over the dish.

4. Place in the oven and bake for 20 minutes. Remove the tray, give it a shake, and return to the oven to bake for another 10 minutes or until the mixture has turned a golden, brown color. Allow to cool, then serve.

Nutrition:

Calories: 241

Fat: 6g

Carbs: 33g

Protein: 15g

14. Med-Styled Olives

Preparation Time: 10 minutes

Cooking Time: 10 minutes

Servings: 6 servings

Ingredients:

- 1 pinch of salt

- 1 pinch of black pepper

- 1 ½ tablespoon of coriander seeds

- 1 tablespoon of extra-virgin olive oil

- 1 lemon

- 7 oz. of kalamata olives

- 7 oz. of green queen olives

Directions:

1. Crush the coriander seeds using your pestle and mortar and set aside. Using a sharp knife, cut long, thin slices of lemon rind and place them into a bowl with both the green queen and kalamata olives.

2. Squeeze the juice of one lemon over the top of the olives and add the olive oil. Add the salt, pepper, and coriander seeds, then stir and serve.

Nutrition:

Calories: 477

Fat: 9g

Carbs: 60g/Protein: 35g

15. Roasted Chickpeas

Preparation Time: 10 minutes

Cooking Time: 40 minutes

Servings: 6 servings

Ingredients:

- 1 pinch of salt

- 1 pinch of black pepper

- 1 pinch of garlic powder

- 1 teaspoon of dried oregano

- 2 tablespoons of extra-virgin olive oil

- juice of 1 lemon

- 2 teaspoons of red wine vinegar

- 2 15 oz. canned chickpeas

Directions:

1. Warm your oven to 425 F and place a sheet of parchment paper onto a baking tray. Drain and rinse

the chickpeas, then pour them onto the baking tray. Spread them evenly.

2. Place them in the oven and roast them for 10 minutes. Remove from the oven, give the plate a firm shake, and then return it to the oven for a further 10 minutes.

3. Remove from the oven and set aside. Add the remaining ingredients into a mixing bowl. Combine well, then add the roasted chickpeas.

4. Using a spatula ensures that the chickpeas are evenly coated. Return the chickpeas into the oven and allow to roast for 10 minutes. Remove them from the oven, allow to cool, then serve.

Nutrition:

Calories: 323

Fat: 15.6g

Carbs: 39.5g

Protein: 10.4g

16. Baked Root Veg Crisps

Preparation Time: 10 minutes

Cooking Time: 30 minutes

Servings: 2

Ingredients:

- 1 pinch of salt

- 1 pinch of black pepper

- 1 pinch of ground cumin

- 1 pinch of dried thyme

- 1 teaspoon of garlic powder

- 2 tablespoons of extra-virgin olive oil

- 1 parsnip, finely sliced

- 1 turnip, finely sliced

- 1 red beet, finely sliced

- 1 golden beet, finely sliced

- Ingredients for the dipping sauce:

- 1 pinch of salt

- 1 pinch of black pepper

- 6 tablespoons of buttermilk

- 1 cup of Greek yogurt

- 1 teaspoon of honey

- 1 teaspoon of lemon zest

- 2 cloves of garlic, minced

- 2 tablespoons of fresh, flat-leaf parsley, minced

Directions:

1. Combine all of the dipping sauce ingredients into a medium mixing bowl, using a whisk to ensure that the sauce is evenly combined. Set aside in the refrigerator for when needed. Preheat your oven to 400 F.

2. In a small mixing bowl, combine the seasoning, herbs, and olive oil. Rinse your root vegetables and dry them off using a kitchen towel.

3. Remove all the root vegetable skins, gently use a mandoline slicer, and slice the vegetables into thin crisps.

4. Brush each side of the crisp with the olive oil and then place onto an oven-proof wire rack. Place the wire rack onto a baking sheet.

5. Bake for 20 minutes or until the vegetables have crisped up. Allow to cool or enjoy them warm with the sauce.

Nutrition:

Calories: 457

Fat: 31g

Carbs: 33g

Protein: 12g

17. Lemon Ricotta Cookies with Lemon Glaze

Preparation Time: 20 minutes

Cooking Time: 15 minutes

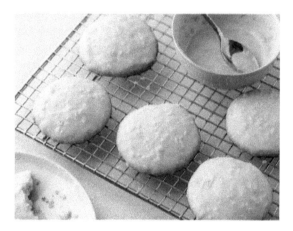

Servings: 44

Ingredients:

- 2 ½ cups all-purpose flour

- 1 tsp baking powder

- 1 tsp salt

- 1 tbsp unsalted butter softened

- 2 cups of sugar

- 2 eggs

- 1 teaspoon (15-ounce) container whole-milk ricotta cheese

- 3 tbsp lemon juice

- zest of one lemon

Glaze:

- 11/2 cups powdered sugar

- 3 tbsp lemon juice

- zest of one lemon

Directions:

1. Warm oven to 375 F. In a medium bowl, combine the flour, baking powder, and salt. Set-aside.

2. From the big bowl, blend the butter and the sugar. With an electric mixer, beat the sugar and butter until light and fluffy, about three minutes. Put the eggs one at a time, beating until incorporated.

3. Insert the ricotta cheese, lemon juice, and lemon zest. Beat to blend. Stir in the dry ingredients — line two baking sheets with parchment paper.

4. Spoon the dough (approximately 2 tablespoons of each cookie) on the baking sheets. Bake within 15 minutes, until slightly golden at the borders. Remove from the oven and allow the cookies to remain on the baking sheet for about 20 minutes.

5. For the glaze, combine the powdered sugar, lemon juice, and lemon zest in a small bowl and then stir until smooth.

6. Spoon approximately 1/2-tsp on each cookie and use the back of the spoon to disperse lightly. Allow glaze to harden for about two hours. Pack the biscuits in a decorative jar.

Nutrition:

Calories: 113

Fat: 3.5 g

Carbs: 19 g

Protein: 0 g

18. Peanut Butter Snack Balls

Preparation Time: 10 minutes

Cooking Time: 0 minutes

Servings: 16

Ingredients:

- 1/2 cup chunky peanut butter

- 3 tbsp flax seeds

- 3 tbsp wheat germ

- 1 tbsp honey or agave

- 1/4 cup powdered sugar

Directions:

1. Blend dry ingredients and adding from honey and peanut butter. Mix well and roll into chunks and then conclude by rolling into wheat germ. Serve.

Nutrition:

Calories: 59

Carbs: 8g

Fat: 2g .Protein: 1g

19. Mascarpone Cheesecake with Almond Crust

Preparation Time: 15 minutes

Cooking Time: 1 hour

Servings: 12

Ingredients:

Crust:

- 1/2 cup slivered almonds

- 8 tsp or 2/3 cup graham cracker crumbs

- 2 tbsp sugar

- 1 tbsp salted butter melted

Filling:

- 1 (8-ounce) packages cream cheese, room temperature

- 1 (8-ounce) container mascarpone cheese, room temperature

- 3/4 cup sugar

- 1 tsp fresh lemon juice

- 1 tsp vanilla extract

- 2 large eggs, room temperature

Directions:

1. For the crust, warm the oven to 350 degrees F. You will need a 9-inch pan. Finely grind the almonds, cracker crumbs sugar in a food processor. Put the butter and process until moist crumbs form.

2. Press the almond mixture on the prepared pan's base (maybe not on the edges of the pan). Bake the crust until it's set and start to brown, about 1-2 minutes. Cool. Adjust the temperature to 325 degrees F.

3. For your filling, with an electric mixer, beat the cream cheese, mascarpone cheese, and sugar in a large bowl until smooth, occasionally scraping down the sides of the jar using a rubber spatula.

4. Beat in the lemon juice and vanilla. Put the eggs one at a time, beating until combined after each addition.

5. Pour the cheese mixture on the crust from the pan. Put the pan into a big skillet or Pyrex dish pour enough hot

water into the roasting pan to come halfway up the sides of one's skillet.

6. Bake until the middle of the filling moves slightly when the pan is gently shaken, about 1 hour. Transfer the cake to a stand; chill for 1 hour. Refrigerate until the cheesecake is cold, at least eight hours.

7. For the topping, squeeze just a small thick cream in the microwave using a chopped Lindt dark chocolate - afterward, get a Ziplock baggie and cut out a hole at the corner, then pour the melted chocolate into the baggie and used this to decorate the cake!

Nutrition:

Calories: 410

Carbs: 39g

Fat: 26g

Protein: 7g

20. Pizza Kale Chips

Preparation Time: 20 minutes

Cooking Time: 12 hours

Servings: 6

Ingredients:

- 1 tsp dried oregano

- 1 tsp dried marjoram

- 1 tsp garlic powder

- 1 tsp onion powder

- 8 cup kale, leaves from about six stalks, veins removed

- 1 cup raw cashew

- 1/2 cup tomato paste, one small can

- 2 tbsp. nutritional yeast, Lewis labs brewer's yeast buds (from sugar beets)

- 1/2 tsp salt

- 1/4 tsp red pepper flakes

- 1 tsp dried basil

- 1/2 tsp dried rosemary

Directions:

1. Place the cashews in a tub, cover with filtered water and allow the cashews, preferably overnight, to soak refrigerated for at least 2 hours.

2. Drain away the cashew juice. Place the cashews in a meal processor or blender. To only cover the cashews, apply filtered water, and heat until creamy smooth.

3. Stir together the cashew cream in a large mixing bowl with all remaining ingredients except the kale. Stir until the combination is even. Rinse the kale and take the leaves off the fibrous roots. Tear the pieces into "chip" size.

4. Take the kale away with the cashew cream filled with "pizza." You may need to do this a little bit at a time, ensuring that coverage is assured. Dehydrate the kale chips for 12 hours, then cook at 105-115 degrees. Serve.

Nutrition:

Calories: 304

Fat: 17 g

Carbs: 27 g

21. Tuscan Bean Stew

Preparation Time: 10 minutes

Cooking Time: 40 minutes

Servings: 4

Ingredients:

- 1 tbsp. extra virgin olive oil

- 50g red onion, finely chopped

- 30g carrot, peeled and finely chopped

- 30g celery, trimmed and finely chopped

- One garlic clove, finely chopped

- ½ bird's eye chili, finely chopped (optional)

- 1 tsp herbs de Provence

- 200ml vegetable stock

- 1 x 400g tin chopped Italian tomatoes

- 1 tsp tomato purée

- 200g tinned mixed beans

- 50g kale, roughly chopped

- 1 tbsp. roughly chopped parsley

- 40g buckwheat

Directions:

1. Put the oil over low to medium heat in a medium saucepan and fry the onion, carrot, celery, garlic, chili, and herbs gently until the onion is soft but not colored.

2. Stir in stock, tomatoes, and purée tomatoes and carry to boil. Attach the beans and require cooking for 30 minutes. Put the kale and cook for within 5–10 minutes, then add the parsley until tender.

3. In the meantime, cook the buckwheat as instructed by the package, drain, and then serve with stew.

Nutrition:

Calories: 365

Fat: 5 g

Carbs: 67 g

Protein: 16 g

22. Chocolate Nut Truffles

Preparation Time: 10 minutes

Cooking Time: 5 minutes

Servings: 25

Ingredients:

- 1 tbsp. Frangelico or 1 tsp vanilla extract

- 50g hazelnut, roughly chopped

- 175ml double cream

- 200g bar dark chocolate, finely chopped

- Different colored sprinkles and edible glitters

Directions:

1. Put the milk into a tiny saucepan to the boiling level. Take the minced chocolate from the flame and pour it over.

2. Gently whisk the mixture up to clear, then apply the alcohol or coffee extract and the hazelnuts. Cover and

put in the fridge for 30 minutes, or until dense but not substantial.

3. Scoop out the mixture's teaspoons and form with your hands into little spheres. Place each of your sprinkles or glitters on different plaques or containers.

4. Roll each truffle to cover in the sprinkles or shimmer, then chill again to firm up. Will keep it refrigerated for one week or freeze without decoration for up to 1 month.

Nutrition:

Calories: 90

Fat: 7 g

Carbs: 5 g

Protein: 1 g

23. Chocolate Balls

Preparation Time: 15 minutes

Cooking Time: 0 minute

Servings: 36

Ingredients:

- 400g can condensed milk

- 1/2 cup desiccated coconut

- 200 grams Arrowroot biscuits crushed

- 3 tablespoons cacao powder

Directions:

1. Mix the broken biscuit, chocolate, and condensed milk to create a sticky consistency. Using a generous mixture tablespoon, shape into balls and wrap in coconut. Chill it before you drink.

Nutrition:

Calories: 121

Fat: 7.8 g

Carbs: 12.9 g .Protein: 2.5 g

24. Vanilla Crème Brule

Preparation Time: 20 minutes

Cooking Time: 30 minutes

Servings: 4

Ingredients:

- 1 cup vanilla sugar, divided

- 6 large egg yolks

- 2 quarts hot water

- 1-quart heavy cream

- 1 vanilla bean split and scraped

Directions:

1. Preheat the oven to 160°C.

2. Place the milk, vanilla bean, and pulp in a medium-high heat saucepan and bring to a boil. Remove from the heat, cover, and allow for 15 minutes of sitting. Remove the vanilla bean and set aside for further use.

3. Whisk 1/2 cup sugar and the egg yolks together in a medium bowl until well mixed until it only begins to lighten in color.

4. Apply the milk, continually mixing, a little at a time. Pour the liquid into six ramekins, then put it in a large cake saucepan or roast pan.

5. Put enough hot water into your saucepan to halfway up the sides of the ramekins. Bake for about 40 to 45 minutes until the crème Brule is set but still trembling in the center.

6. Remove the ramekins from the roasting oven, and cool for at least two hours and up to three days in general.

7. Reserve the Brule cream from the refrigerator for at least 30 minutes before the sugar has browned. Divide the remaining 1/2 cup vanilla sugar equally over the six bowls, then sprinkle uniformly over the bottom.

8. Melt the sugar using a flame, then shape a crispy layer. Enable the crème Brule to sit for 5 minutes or more before serving.

Nutrition:

Calories: 400

Carbs: 26 g

Fat: 32 g

Protein: 3 g

25. Healthy Coffee Cookies

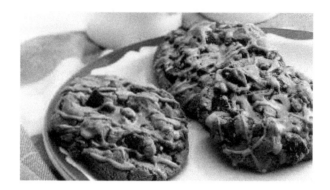

Preparation time: 15 – 20 minutes

Cooking time: 12 - 15 minutes

Servings: 20

Ingredients:

For dry ingredients:

- ½ cup cocoa, unsweetened

- 6 tablespoons all-purpose flour

- ½ cup whole-wheat flour

- ¾ tablespoon finely ground coffee beans or instant coffee

- ½ teaspoon baking soda

- ¾ teaspoon ground cinnamon

- ¼ teaspoon kosher salt

For wet ingredients:

- 3 small eggs, lightly beaten

- ¼ cup nonfat or low-fat plain Greek yogurt

- ½ tablespoon olive oil

- ½ + 1/8 cup blueberries

- ½ ripe banana

- ¼ cup honey

- 1 teaspoon pure vanilla extract

- ¼ cup dark or semi-sweet chocolate chips

Directions:

1. Preheat the oven to 350°F. Prepare a baking sheet by oiling with nonstick cooking spray. Set it aside.

2. Combine all the dry ingredients, i.e., whole-wheat flour, all-purpose flour, cocoa, cinnamon, salt, baking soda, and coffee in a mixing bowl.

3. Place banana in a microwave-safe bowl and cook on high for about 50 seconds. Mash the banana and add

into a bowl. Also, add eggs, yogurt, oil, honey, and vanilla. Mix until well incorporated.

4. Pour the wet ingredients into the dry ingredients and mix until just combined, making sure not to over-mix. Add chocolate chips and blueberries and fold gently.

5. Make 20 equal portions of the mixture and place it on the baking sheet. It should be approximately 1-½ tablespoons per portion. Press the cookies lightly. You can use a fork to do so.

6. Put the baking sheet in your oven and bake within about 12 – 14 minutes. When the cookies are ready, they will be visibly hard around the edges.

7. Cool on the baking sheet for 10 minutes. Loosen the cookies by pushing a metal spatula underneath the cookies. Transfer onto a wire rack. Serve.

Nutrition:

Calories 60

Fat 1.5 g

Carbohydrate 11 g

Protein 2 g

26. Strawberry Oatmeal Bars

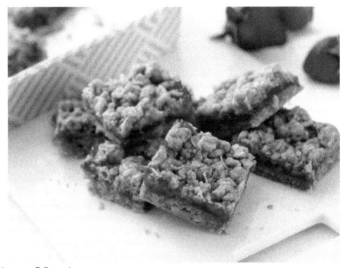

Preparation time: 20 minutes

Cooking time: 35 – 40 minutes

Servings: 8

Ingredients:

For strawberry bars:

- ½ cup old-fashioned rolled oats

- 3 tablespoons light brown sugar

- 1/8 teaspoon kosher salt

- 1 cup small-diced strawberries, divided

- ½ tablespoon fresh lemon juice

- 6 tablespoons white whole wheat flour

- 1/8 teaspoon ground ginger

- 3 tablespoons unsalted butter, melted

- ½ teaspoon cornstarch

- 3 teaspoons granulated sugar, divided

For the vanilla glaze: Optional

- ¼ cup powdered sugar sifted

- ½ tablespoon milk

- ¼ teaspoon pure vanilla extract

Directions:

1. Preheat the oven to 350°F. Prepare a small square or rectangular baking pan by lining it with a large parchment paper sheet such that the extra sheet is hanging from 2 opposite sides.

2. Add oats, brown sugar, flour, salt, and ginger into a bowl and stir well. Put butter and mix.

3. Take out about 4 tablespoons of the mixture into a bowl and set it aside. Transfer the rest of the mixture into the baking pan. Press it well onto the bottom of the baking pan.

4. Spread ½ cup chopped strawberries over the crust — dust cornstarch over it. Drizzle the lemon juice over the strawberries. Sprinkle 1 ½ teaspoons sugar.

5. Spread remaining strawberries and 1 ½ teaspoons sugar over it. Scatter the retained crumb mixture on top. Put the baking dish in your oven and bake for about 30 – 35 minutes or until golden brown on top. Take out the baking dish and place it on the wire rack to cool.

6. Meanwhile, make the glaze. For this, add powdered sugar, milk, and vanilla into a bowl and whisk well. Lift the bars along with the parchment paper and place it on your cutting board. Pour glaze on top. Cut into 8 equal bars and serve.

Nutrition:

Calories 100

Fat 5 g

Carbohydrate 14 gProtein 2 g

27. Parsley Cheese Balls

Preparation time: 15 minutes

Cooking time: 0 minutes

Servings: 12

Ingredients:

- ¼ cup shredded, Kraft 2% milk sharp cheddar cheese

- 1 package (8 ounces) Philadelphia Neufchatel cheese, softened

- ½ tablespoon finely chopped green onion

- ½ tablespoon finely chopped red pepper

- ¼ cup finely chopped parsley

- 1 teaspoon Dijon mustard

- 6 stalks celery, cut each into 4 equal pieces crosswise

- 60 whole-wheat Ritz crackers

Directions:

1. Add Neufchatel and cheddar cheeses into a bowl. Beat with an electric hand mixer until well combined. Stir in green onion, red pepper, and Dijon mustard.

2. Place the bowl in the refrigerator for an hour. Split the batter into 12 equal portions and shape into balls.

3. Place parsley on a plate. Dredge the balls in parsley. Place on a plate. Chill until use. Each serving should consist of a cheese ball with 2 pieces parsley and 5 Ritz crackers.

Nutrition:

Calories 130

Fat 7 g

Carbohydrate 12 g

Protein 3 g

28. Baked Kale Chips

Preparation time: 10 minutes

Cooking time: 10 minutes

Servings: 3

Ingredients:

- ½ bunch kale (stiff stems and ribs discarded), torn into bite-size pieces

- Salt to taste

- ½ tablespoon olive oil

- Spices of your choice to flavor (optional)

Directions:

1. Preheat the oven to 350°F. Dry the kale using a salad spinner. Place kale on the baking sheet. Trickle oil over it. Sprinkle salt over the kale and spread it evenly.

2. Put the baking sheet in your oven and bake within about 12 – 14 minutes or until crisp. Cool completely and serve. Store the leftovers in an airtight container.

Nutrition:

Calories 58

Fat 2.8 g

Carbohydrate 7.6 g

Protein 2.5 g

Chapter 2. Sauces & Dips

29. Sweet and Savory Cherry Compote

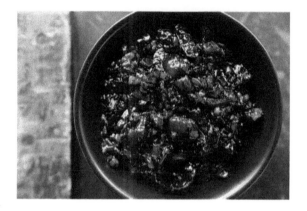

Preparation time: 15 minutes

Cooking time: 10 minutes

Servings: 6

Ingredients:

- 2 1/2 cups pitted sweet cherries, slice into quarter

- 1 cup walnuts, thinly chopped

- 2 tablespoons red onion, diced

- 3 tablespoons extra virgin olive oil

- ¼ cup port red wine or cherry juice

- ¼ tsp sea salt

- 1 tablespoon honey

- 1 teaspoon rosemary, fresh

- ¼ tsp black pepper, ground

Directions:

1. Add the extra virgin olive oil into a large skillet and sauté the red onion over medium heat until the red onion is soft and tender and beginning to turn golden around the edges, about 3 minutes. Be sure to stir the onions occasionally, so the onion cooks evenly.

2. Add the cherries, walnuts, and rosemary to the skillet and continue to stir until the cherries become tender about 5 minutes. Add in the seasonings and adjust the amount to fit your taste.

3. Pour in the red wine or cherry juice along with the honey. Allow the cherries to cook in the wine simmering until the cherries are soft and the liquid has become thick with a syrup-like texture.

Nutrition:

Calories: 120

Carbs: 21g

Fat: 3g

Protein: 3g

30. Cilantro Lime Sauce

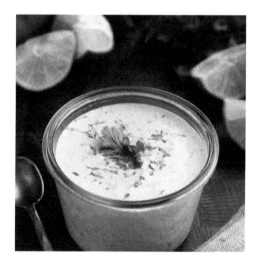

Preparation time: 15 minutes

Cooking time: 0 minutes

Servings: 2

Ingredients:

- ½ cup Soy yogurt, plain

- ½ tsp Black pepper, ground

- 1 tablespoon Lime juice

- 1 teaspoon Lime Zest

- 6 tablespoons cilantro, chopped

- ½ tbsp Extra virgin olive oil

- ½ tsp Sea salt

Directions:

1. Puree all of the cilantro-lime sauce ingredients in a blender or food processor until smooth. Serve the sauce immediately, or store in the fridge for up to a week.

Nutrition:

Calories: 95

Carbs: 1g

Fat: 10g

Protein: 0g

31. Greek Tzatziki Sauce

Preparation time: 15 minutes

Cooking time: 0 minutes

Servings: 12

Ingredients:

- 1 cup Soy yogurt, plain

- 1 & ½ cup English cucumber, grated

- 1 tablespoon Extra virgin olive oil

- 2 cloves garlic, minced

- 2 teaspoons Lemon juice

- ½ tsp Sea salt

- 2 teaspoons parsley, chopped

- 2 teaspoons Dill, chopped

Directions:

1. In a kitchen, a bowl whisks together all of the ingredients, excluding the cucumber. Put the grated

cucumber in a clean towel, and squeeze it over the sink to remove as much liquid as possible.

2. Add the cucumber to the bowl, stirring it together to combine. Serve immediately, or store in the fridge for up to four to five days.

Nutrition:

Calories: 25

Carbs: 3g

Fat: 0g

32. Green Enchilada Sauce

Preparation time: 15 minutes

Cooking time: 12 minutes

Servings: 6

Ingredients:

- ½ cup of water

- ½ cup cashews, raw

- 2 cups cilantro, chopped

- 1 jalapeno, chopped

- 7 oz green chilies, canned

- 1 & ½ tsp apple cider vinegar

- 1 teaspoon of sea salt

Directions:

1. Soak or dip the cashews, cover them with water and allow them to sit covered for 6 to 12 hours, or simmer

them on the stove in water for 15 minutes. Drain off the water and add the cashews to a blender.

2. Into the blender, add the remaining ingredients, and blend the enchilada sauce until it is completely smooth. Use the green enchilada sauce immediately or store it in the refrigerator for up to a week.

Nutrition:

Calories: 25

Carbs: 3g

Fat: 2g

33. Jalapeno Pineapple Aioli

Preparation time: 15 minutes

Cooking time: 0 minutes

Servings: 12

Ingredients:

- 1 1/2 cups mayonnaise made with olive oil

- 3 tablespoons onion, minced

- ¼ cup cilantro, chopped

- 1 jalapeno, minced

- ½ cup canned pineapple, minced

- 1 clove garlic, minced

- 2 tablespoons pineapple juice from the can

- 1 tablespoon lime juice

- ½ tsp sea salt

- ½ tsp red pepper flakes

- 1 teaspoon lime zest

Directions:

1. If you want a chunky sauce, add everything to a bowl and stir it. For a smooth, creamy sauce, pulse everything together in a blender until creamy. Serve the jalapeno pineapple aioli immediately or store in the fridge for up to a week.

Nutrition:

Calories: 172

Carbs: 6g

Fat: 16g

Protein: 1g

34. Awesome Sauce

Preparation time: 15 minutes

Cooking time: 3 minutes

Servings: 8

Ingredients:

- ½ cup Mayonnaise made with olive oil

- 1 teaspoon Sea salt

- 2 teaspoons Mustard

- 1 cup Onion, diced

- 1 tablespoon Extra virgin olive oil

- 2 tablespoons parsley, chopped

- 1 tablespoon Chives, chopped

- 1 tablespoon Dill, chopped

- ¼ tsp Black pepper, ground

Directions:

1. Add the onions and olive oil to a skillet, allowing them to sauté until slightly translucent, about three minutes over medium-high heat.

2. In a blender, combine all of the awesome sauce ingredients, except for the chopped herbs. Continue to pulse until creamy, and then gently stir in the chopped herbs. Serve the sauce immediately, or store in the fridge for up to a week.

Nutrition:

Calories: 80

Carbs: 1g

Fat: 7g

Protein: 0g

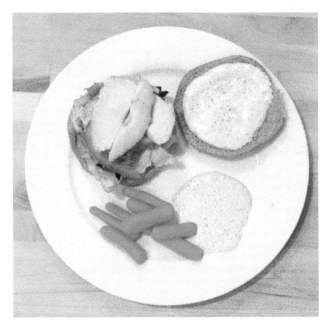

35. Vegan Hollandaise Sauce

Preparation time: 15 minutes

Cooking time: 0 minutes

Servings: 8

Ingredients:

- 1 cup Mayonnaise made with olive oil (vegan)

- 1 teaspoon Lemon juice

- 3 tablespoons vegan butter, melted

- ½ tsp Turmeric, ground

- ¼ tsp Cayenne pepper

- ¼ tsp Black pepper, ground

Directions:

1. Add all of the vegan Hollandaise sauce ingredients to a small saucepan and cook it over medium heat until heated through. Be careful not to allow the Hollandaise sauce to boil. Remove from heat and use hot. Enjoy the sauce immediately, or store it for up to a week.

Nutrition:

Calories: 67

Carbs: 0g Fat: 7g Protein: 1g

36. Vegan Cheese Sauce

Preparation time: 15 minutes

Cooking time: 10 minutes

Servings: 6

Ingredients:

- 1 yellow summer squash, sliced

- 1 sweet potato, medium, peeled and diced

- 4 cloves garlic, minced

- 1 onion, diced

- 2 cups vegetable broth

- ¼ cup nutritional yeast

- 1 & ½ tsp sea salt

- ¼ tsp mustard powder

- ¼ tsp paprika

- ¼ tsp black pepper, ground

Directions:

1. Add the diced potato to a pot of boiling water, and allow it to cook until tender, about seven to ten minutes.

2. Meanwhile, sauté the onion and yellow squash in the vegetable broth. Slowly add the vegetable broth as needed, using about one-quarter of a cup at a time and adding more as needed.

3. Add in the minced garlic, and sauté until it becomes aromatic about 3 minutes. Add the cooked onion, squash, and potato into a blender with the remaining vegetable broth and all of the seasonings.

4. Combine at high speed until the sauce is incredibly smooth. Feel free to add more broth to adjust the thickness to your preference.

Nutrition:

Calories: 37

Carbs: 6g

Fat: 1g

Protein: 3g

37. Teriyaki Sauce

Preparation time: 15 minutes

Cooking time: 5 minutes

Servings: 6

Ingredients:

- ¼ cup tamari sauce

- 1 & ¼ cup water, divided

- 2 tablespoons cornstarch

- ¼ cup honey

- ½ tsp ginger, grated

- 1 clove garlic, minced

Directions:

1. Mix the one-quarter cup of water and cornstarch in a small bowl. Set the slurry aside.

2. In a saucepan, add the remaining water and the tamari sauce, honey, garlic, and ginger. While stirring, cook over medium heat until it reaches a simmer.

3. Add the cornstarch slurry into the saucepan while whisking, and continue to cook the sauce until thickened, about seven minutes.

4. Remove the easy teriyaki sauce from the stove and allow it to sit for five to ten minutes before using, to let it to finish thickening.

Nutrition:

Calories: 15

Carbs: 2g

Fat: 0g

Protein: 1g

38. Thai Peanut Sauce

Preparation time: 15 minutes

Cooking time: 0 minutes

Servings: 6

Ingredients:

- ½ cup peanut butter, natural

- 1 teaspoon honey

- ½ cup of soy milk

- 2 tablespoons tamari sauce

- ½ tsp ginger, grated

- 1 tablespoon lime juice

- 1 teaspoon sriracha sauce

- 1 clove garlic, minced

Directions:

1. Add all of the Thai peanut sauce ingredients into a blender and combine until smooth, and the garlic is

well combined. Use the peanut sauce immediately or store it in the fridge for up to a week.

Nutrition:

Calories: 40

Carbs: 3g

Fat: 2g

Protein: 1g

39. Tasty Vegan Gravy

Preparation time: 15 minutes

Cooking time: 17 minutes

Servings: 6

Ingredients:

- 2 cloves garlic, minced

- ½ tsp sea salt

- 4 ounces mushrooms, sliced

- 1 onion, diced

- 1 tablespoon extra-virgin olive oil

- 1 Yukon gold potato, peeled and diced

- 1 cup of water

- 2 tablespoons tamari sauce

- ¼ tsp black pepper, ground

Directions:

1. Sauté your onion in the extra virgin olive oil until tender and translucent, about 5 minutes, and then add in the mushrooms and garlic. Continue stirring until the garlic is fragrant and golden, about 1 to 2 minutes.

2. Into the skillet, add the Yukon Gold potato, water, and tamari sauce, allowing it to reach a boil over medium-high heat.

3. Reduce the stove to medium and cover the steel skillet with a lid. Allow the potatoes to cook until they are tender, about 10 minutes.

4. Carefully pour the potatoes, mushrooms, and other skillet contents into a blender along with the seasonings.

5. Instead of the plastic cap, use a towel to cover the opening, which will allow steam to escape while also keeping the contents in the blender.

6. Blend the contents at high speed until completely smooth and creamy. Adjust the seasoning to your taste and enjoy.

Nutrition:

Calories: 31

Carbs: 6g

Fat: 0g

Protein: 2g

Chapter 3. Juices & Smoothies

40. Kale Kiwi Smoothie

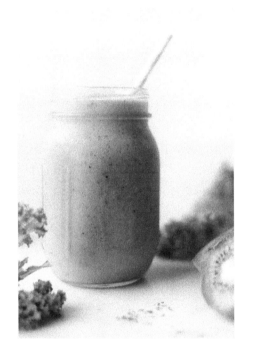

Preparation Time: 10 minutes

Cooking Time: 0 minutes

Servings: 1

Ingredients:

- 1 cup kale, chopped

- 2 Apples

- 3 Kiwis

- 1 tablespoon flax seeds

- 1 tablespoon royal jelly

- 1 cup crushed ice

Directions:

1. Put all of the fixings into a blender and cover them with water. Blitz until smooth. Serve.

Nutrition:

Calories: 250

Carbs: 35g

Fat: 1g

Protein: 15g

41. Salad Smoothie

Preparation Time: 10 minutes

Cooking Time: 0 minutes

Servings: 1

Ingredients:

- 1 cup arugula

- ½ cucumber

- 1/2 small red onion

- 2 tablespoons Parsley

- 2 tablespoons lemon juice

- 1 cup crushed ice

- 1 tbsp. olive oil or cumin oil

Directions:

1. Put all the fixing into a blender with some water and blitz until smooth. Add ice to make your smoothie refreshing.

Nutrition:

Calories: 80

Carbs: 20g

Fat: 0g

Protein: 1g

42. Avocado Kale Smoothie

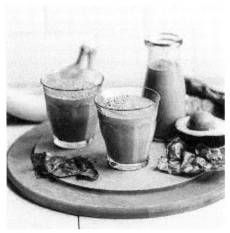

Preparation Time: 10 minutes

Cooking Time: 0 minutes

Servings: 1

Ingredients:

- 1 cup kale

- ½ avocado

- 1 cup cucumber

- 1 celery stalk

- 1 tbsp. chia seeds

- 1 cup crushed ice

- 1 tbsp. spirulina

Directions:

1. Put all of the fixings into a blender and add in enough water to cover them. Process until smooth, serve, and enjoy.

Nutrition:

Calories: 377

Carbs: 0g

Fat: 0g

Protein: 0g

43. Kale Banana Apple Smoothie

Preparation Time: 10 minutes

Cooking Time: 0 minutes

Servings: 1

Ingredients:

- 1 cup kale

- 2 apples

- 3/4 avocado

- 1 banana

- 1 cup crushed ice

Directions:

1. Put all of the fixings into a blender and process until smooth. Serve and enjoy.

Nutrition:

Calories: 150

Carbs: 29g

Fat: 0g

Protein: 2g

44. Kale Cucumber Apple Smoothie

Preparation Time: 10 minutes

Cooking Time: 0 minutes

Servings: 1

Ingredients:

- 1 cup kale

- 2 apples

- 1 avocado

- 1 lime

- 1/4 cup raspberries

- 1 cucumber

- 1 cup crushed ice

Directions:

1. Put all of the fixings into the blender with enough water to cover them and blitz until smooth.

Nutrition:

Calories: 120

Carbs: 0g

Fat: 0g

Protein: 5g

45. Grapefruit Kale Smoothie

Preparation Time: 10 minutes

Cooking Time: 0 minutes

Servings: 1

Ingredients:

- 1 large grapefruit

- 1 apple

- 1 cup watercress

- 2 kale leaves

- 1 tbsp. dill (optional)

- 1 cup crushed ice

Directions:

1. Put all of the fixings into a blender and add enough water to cover them. Process until creamy and smooth.

Nutrition:

Calories: 233

Carbs: 37g

Fat: 4g .Protein: 16g

46. Pear Cilantro Smoothie

Preparation Time: 10 minutes

Cooking Time: 0 minutes

Servings: 1

Ingredients:

- 1 cup parsley leaves

- 1 pear

- 3/4 avocado

- ½ lemon - juice

- 1 tbsp. chopped cilantro

- 1 cup crushed ice

Directions:

1. Process all of the fixings into a blender with water to cover them. Add a few ice cubes and enjoy.

Nutrition:

Calories: 413

Carbs: 97g .Fat: 3g .Protein: 3g

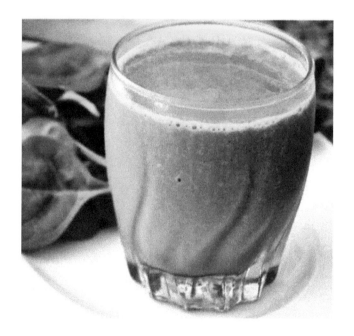

47. Kefir Kale Banana Orange Chia Smoothie

Preparation Time: 10 minutes

Cooking Time: 0 minutes

Servings: 1

Ingredients:

- 1/2 orange

- 1 banana

- 1 cup kale

- 1/4 cup chia seeds

- 1/2 cup kefir

- 1 cup crushed ice

Directions:

1. Put all of the fixings into a blender with enough water to cover them and process until smooth. Add a few ice cubes and enjoy.

Nutrition:

Calories: 214

Carbs: 45g

Fat: 0g

Protein: 2g

48. Matcha Apple & Greens Juice

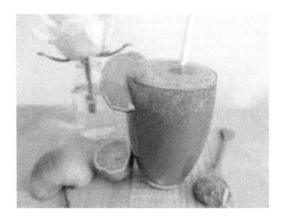

Preparation Time: 10 minutes

Cooking Time: 0 minutes

Servings: 2

Ingredients:

- 5 ounces fresh kale

- 2 ounces fresh arugula

- ¼ cup fresh parsley

- 4 celery stalks

- 1 green apple, cored and chopped

- 1 (1-inch) piece fresh ginger, peeled

- 1 lemon, peeled

- ½ teaspoon matcha green tea

Directions:

1. Add all kale, arugula, green apple, and other fixings into a juicer and extract. Pour into 2 glasses and serve immediately.

Nutrition:

Calories 113

Fat 0.6 g

Carbs 26.7 g

Protein 3.8 g

49. Celery Juice

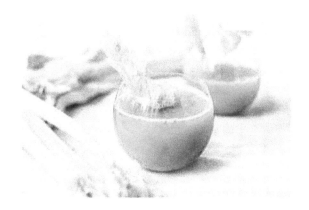

Preparation Time: 10 minutes

Cooking Time: 0 minutes

Servings: 2

Ingredients:

- 8 celery stalks with leaves

- 2 tablespoons fresh ginger, peeled

- 1 lemon, peeled

- ½ cup of filtered water

- Pinch of salt

Directions:

1. Pulse all the fixing in a blender. Strain the juice and transfer it into two glasses. Serve immediately.

Nutrition:

Calories 32

Fat 0.5 g

Carbs 6.5 g

Protein 1 g

50. Apple, Cucumber & Celery Juice

Preparation Time: 10 minutes

Cooking Time: 0 minutes

Servings: 2

Ingredients:

- 3 large apples, cored and sliced

- 2 large cucumbers, sliced

- 4 celery stalks

- 1 (1-inch) piece fresh ginger, peeled

- 1 lemon, peeled

Directions:

1. Add apples, cucumber, and others into a juicer, then extract. Pour into two glasses and serve immediately.

Nutrition:

Calories 230

Fat 1.1 g Carbs 59.5 g .Protein 3.3 g

51. Lemony Apple & Kale Juice

Preparation Time: 10 minutes

Cooking Time: 0 minutes

Servings: 2

Ingredients:

- 2 large green apples, cored and sliced

- 4 cups fresh kale leaves

- 4 tablespoons fresh parsley leaves

- 1 tablespoon fresh ginger, peeled

- 1 lemon, peeled

- ½ cup of filtered water

- Pinch of salt

Directions:

1. Pulse all the fixing in a blender well combined. the juice and transfer it glasses.

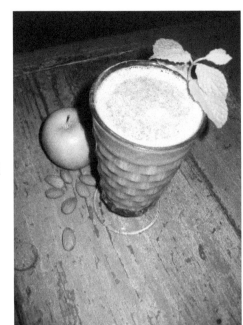

listed until Strain into 2 Serve.

Nutrition:

Calories 196

Fat 0.6 g

Carbs 47.9 g

52. Orange Juice

Preparation time: 10 minutes

Cooking time: 0 minutes

Servings: 2

Ingredients:

- 5 large oranges, peeled and portioned

Directions:

1. Add all ingredients into a juicer and extract the juice. Pour into 2 glasses and serve immediately.

Nutrition:

Calories: 45

Carbs: 10g

Fat: 0g

Protein: 1g

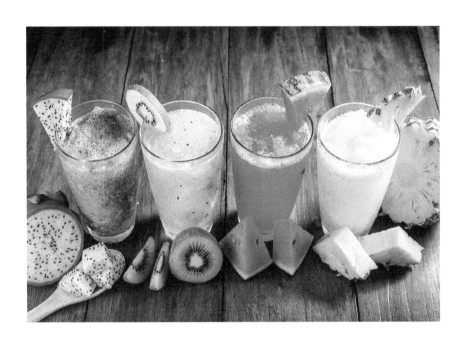

53. Apple & Cucumber Juice

Preparation time: 10 minutes

Cooking time: 0 minutes

Servings: 2

Ingredients:

- 3 large apples, cored and sliced

- 2 large cucumbers, sliced

- 4 celery stalks

- 1 (1-inch) piece fresh ginger, peeled

- 1 lemon, peeled

Directions:

1. Extract all listed fixing into a juicer. Pour into 2 glasses and serve.

Nutrition:

Calories: 80

Carbs: 20g

Fat: 0g .Protein: 3g

54. Apple & Celery Juice

Preparation Time: 10 minutes

Cooking Time: 0 minutes

Servings: 2

Ingredients:

- 4 large green apples, cored and sliced

- 4 large celery stalks

- 1 lemon, peeled

Directions:

1. Add green apples, celery stalks, and lemon into a juicer and extract. Pour into two glasses and serve immediately.

Nutrition:

Calories 240

Fat 0.9g

Carbs 63.3 g

Protein 1.5 g

55. Apple, Orange & Broccoli Juice

Preparation Time: 10 minutes

Cooking Time: 0 minutes

Servings: 2

Ingredients:

- 2 broccoli stalks, chopped

- 2 large green apples, cored and sliced

- 3 large oranges, peeled and sectioned

- 4 tablespoons fresh parsley

Directions:

1. Add all fixing into a juicer and extract. Pour into your glasses and serve immediately.

Nutrition:

Calories 254

Fat 0.8 g

Carbs 64.7 g Protein 3.8 g

56. Apple, Grapefruit & Carrot Juice

Preparation Time: 10 minutes

Cooking Time: 0 minutes

Servings: 2

Ingredients:

- 3 cups fresh kale

- 2 large apples, cored and sliced

- 2 medium carrots, peeled and chopped

- 2 medium grapefruit, peeled and sectioned

- 1 teaspoon fresh lemon juice

Directions:

1. Add kale, apples, carrots, and other fixing into a juicer and extract. Pour into two glasses and serve.

Nutrition:

Calories 232

Fat 0.6 g

Carbs 57.7 g

Protein 4.9g

57. Green Fruit Juice

Preparation Time: 10 minutes

Cooking Time: 0 minutes

Servings: 2

Ingredients:

- 3 large kiwis, peeled and chopped

- 3 large green apples, cored and sliced

- 2 cups seedless green grapes

- 2 teaspoons fresh lime juice

Directions:

1. Add kiwis, apples, grapes, and lime juice into a juicer and extract. Pour into 2 glasses, then serve immediately.

Nutrition:

Calories 304

Fat 2.2 g Carbs 79 g Protein 6.2 g

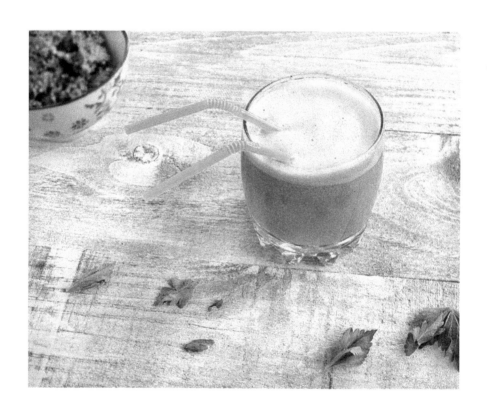

58. Apple & Carrot Juice

Preparation Time: 10 minutes

Cooking Time: 0 minutes

Servings: 2

Ingredients:

- 5 carrots, peeled and chopped

- 1 large apple, cored and chopped

- 1 (½-inch) piece fresh ginger, peeled and chopped

- ½ of lemon

Directions:

1. Add carrots, apple, ginger, and lemon into a juicer, then extract. Pour into two glasses and serve immediately.

Nutrition:

Calories 125

Fat 0.3 g

Carbs 31.4 g

Protein 1.7 g

59. Lemony Green Juice

Preparation time: 10 minutes

Cooking time: 0 minutes

Servings: 2

Ingredients:

- 2 large green apples, cored and sliced

- 4 cups fresh kale leaves

- 4 tablespoons fresh parsley leaves

- 1 tablespoon fresh ginger, peeled

- 1 lemon, peeled

- ½ cup of filtered water

- Pinch of salt

Directions:

1. Put all the fixing in a blender and pulse until well combined. Strain the juice, then transfer into 2 glasses. Serve immediately.

Nutrition:

Calories: 110

Carbs: 25g

Fat: 1g

Protein: 5g

60. Sirtfood Smoothie

Preparation time: 15 minutes

Cooking time: 0 minutes

Servings: 1

Ingredients:

- 3/8 cup of Greek yogurt

- 6 walnut halves

- 10 hulled strawberries

- 7 – 10 kale leaves

- ¾ oz. dark chocolate

- 1 Medjool date

- ½ tsp. ground turmeric

- 1 sliver of Thai chili

- 200ml of unsweetened almond milk

Directions:

1. Load up all the ingredients into your blender and grind into a smooth pulp.

Nutrition:

Calories: 90

Carbs: 20g

Fat: 1g

Protein: 3g

61. Strawberry Juice

Preparation Time: 10 minutes

Cooking Time: 0 minutes

Servings: 2

Ingredients:

- 2½ cups fresh ripe strawberries, hulled

- 1 apple, cored and chopped

- 1 lime, peeled

Directions:

1. Extract all the fixing into a juicer. Pour into two glasses and serve immediately.

Nutrition:

Calories 118

Fat 0.8 g

Carbs 30.1 g

Protein 1.6 g

62. Chocolate Date Smoothie

Preparation Time: 10 minutes

Cooking Time: 0 minutes

Servings: 2

Ingredients:

- 4-5 Medjool dates, pitted

- 2 tablespoons cacao powder

- 2 tablespoons flaxseed

- 1 tablespoon almond butter

- 1 teaspoon vanilla extract

- ¼ teaspoon ground cinnamon

- 1½ cups unsweetened almond milk

- 4 ice cubes

Directions:

1. Add all fixing to a high-power blender and pulse until smooth. Pour into two glasses and serve immediately.

Nutrition:

Calories 264

Fat 10.3 g

Carbs 41.8 g

Protein 6.4 g

63. Blueberry & Kale Smoothie

Preparation Time: 10 minutes

Cooking Time: 0 minutes

Servings: 2

Ingredients:

- 2 cups frozen blueberries

- 2 cups fresh kale leaves

- 2 Medjool dates, pitted

- 1 tablespoon chia seeds

- 2 teaspoons fresh ginger, chopped

- 1½ cups unsweetened almond milk

Directions:

1. Pulse all fixing to your blender until smooth. Serve immediately.

Nutrition:

Calories 230

Fat 4.5 g Carbs 48.8 g Protein 5.6 g

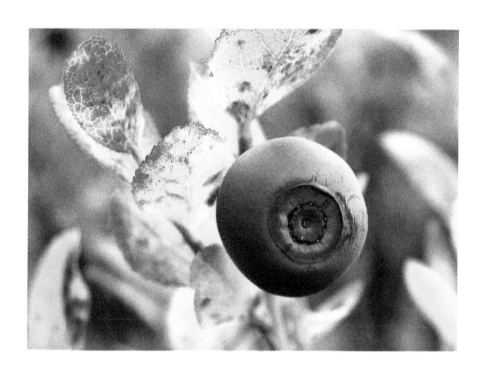

64. Strawberry & Beet Smoothie

Preparation Time: 10 minutes

Cooking Time: 0 minutes

Servings: 2

Ingredients:

- 2 cups frozen strawberries, pitted and chopped

- 2/3 cup frozen beets, chopped

- 1 teaspoon fresh ginger, peeled and chopped

- 1 teaspoon fresh turmeric, peeled and grated

- ½ cup fresh orange juice

- 1 cup unsweetened almond milk

Directions:

1. Blend all the fixing. Serve immediately.

Nutrition:

Calories 130

Fat 2.1 g

Carbs 27.5 g

Protein 2 g

65. Green Pineapple Smoothie

Preparation Time: 5 minutes

Cooking Time: 0 minutes

Servings: 1

Ingredients:

- 50 grams of chard

- 1 apple

- 200 grams of pineapple

- 1tsp. of flax seeds

Directions:

1. All to the glass of the blender with a little water and grind well. Serve.

Nutrition:

Calories 251.16

Carbohydrates 46.44

Proteins 3.51 Fat 4.11

66. Mango Smoothie

Preparation Time: 5 minutes

Cooking Time: 0 minutes

Servings: 1

Ingredients:

- 1 small mango

- 1 hand spinach

- 10 leaves of minutest

- 1/3 avocado

- 1 tbsp. (raw) honey

- 200 ml of water

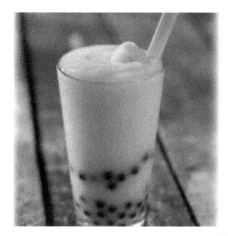

Directions:

1. Get a blender; pour all the ingredients into it, and then blend. Serve.

Nutrition:

Calories 150 Protein 9gFats 0gCarbohydrates 0g

67. Red Wine Hot Chocolate

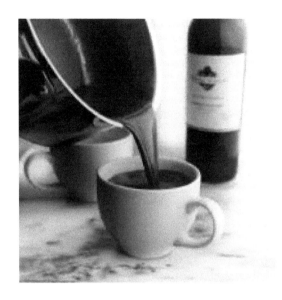

Preparation time: 15 minutes

Cooking time: 5 minutes

Servings: 4

Ingredients:

- 2/3 cup dry red wine

- 2/3 cup semi-sweet chocolate chips

- 2 tbsp. sugar

- ½ cup half and half

- ½ cup milk

- ½ tsp. vanilla extract

- 1/8 tsp. salt

Directions:

1. Set over medium-low heat in a small saucepan, combine wine, chocolate chips, half and half, milk, and sugar; heat, stirring, for about 5 minutes or until chocolate is completely melted. Remove from heat and stir in salt and vanilla; pour into serving mugs and enjoy!

Nutrition:

Calories: 256

Carbs: 39g

Fat: 7g

Protein: 3g

68. Citric Blueberry Slush

Preparation time: 15 minutes

Cooking time: 0 minutes

Servings: 6

Ingredients:

- 1-1/2 cups frozen blueberries

- 1-1/2 cups fresh orange juice

- 2 tbsp. lime juice

- 2 tbsp. lemon juice

- 1/2 cup raw honey

- 1 cup crushed ice

Directions:

1. In a blender, combine honey, lime, lemon, and orange juices; blend until honey is dissolved; add ice cubes and blueberries and puree. Pour into glasses, then garnish with a lime or lemon wedge. Enjoy!

Nutrition:

Calories: 90 Carbs: 27g Fat: 0g .Protein: 0g

69. Citrus, Blueberry & Rosemary Mocktail

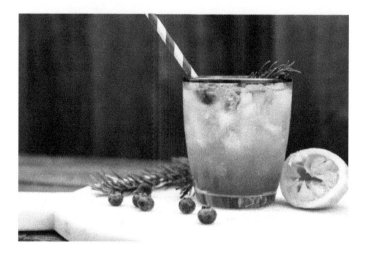

Preparation time: 15 minutes

Cooking time: 10 minutes

Servings: 1

Ingredients:

For rosemary syrup:

- 4 springs fresh rosemary

- ¼ cup of water

- ½ cup of sugar

For cocktail:

- ½ ounce fresh lime juice

- o ounces rosemary syrup

- crushed ice

- Lime slice & fresh blueberries

Directions:

1. For the syrup, combine water, sugar, and rosemary in a pan; simmer for about 10 minutes or until sugar is completely dissolved. Cover the pan and steep within 1 hour.

2. For the mocktail, combine lime juice and rosemary syrup in a shaker and shake to mix well. Pour into serving glasses and stir in ice cubes. Garnish with fresh blueberries and lime slices.

Nutrition:

Calories: 90

Carbs: 19g

Fat: 1g

Protein: 1g

70. Spiced Green Tea Tonic

Preparation time: 15 minutes

Cooking time: 0 minutes

Servings: 1

Ingredients:

- 8 ounces purified water, boiling

- 1 fresh ginger, minced

- 1 bag green tea

- 1/4 tsp. cinnamon

- 1/4 tsp. turmeric

- 1 tbsp. raw honey

Directions

1. Combine the teabag, ginger, and spices in a teacup; add hot water, and follow the package directions to steep the tea. Discard the teabag and stir the mixture to dissolve the spices. Stir in raw honey and serve hot.

Nutrition:

Calories: 82

Carbs: 21g

Fat: 0g .Protein: 1g

71. Green Tea Smoothie

Preparation time: 15 minutes

Cooking time: 0 minutes

Servings: 2

Ingredients:

- 1 cup green tea, brewed, chilled
- 1/4 cup fresh blueberries
- 1/4 cup fresh raspberries
- 1 tbsp. nonfat plain Greek yogurt
- 1 handful of ice cubes

Directions:

1. Combine all fixings in a blender and blend until smooth. Enjoy!

Nutrition:

Calories: 300

Carbs: 50g

Fat: 5g .Protein: 20g

72. Mint, Lemon, and Blueberry Infused Water

Preparation time: 15 minutes

Cooking time: 0 minutes

Servings: 2

Ingredients:

- ½ cup blueberries

- 1 lemon, sliced

- ½ cup chopped mint leaves

- 1 cup of filtered water

Directions

1. In a jar, combine water, blueberries, mint leaves, lemon slices; steep in the refrigerator for at least 3 hours. Enjoy!

Nutrition:

Calories: 10 Carbs: 2g Fat: 0g Protein: 0g

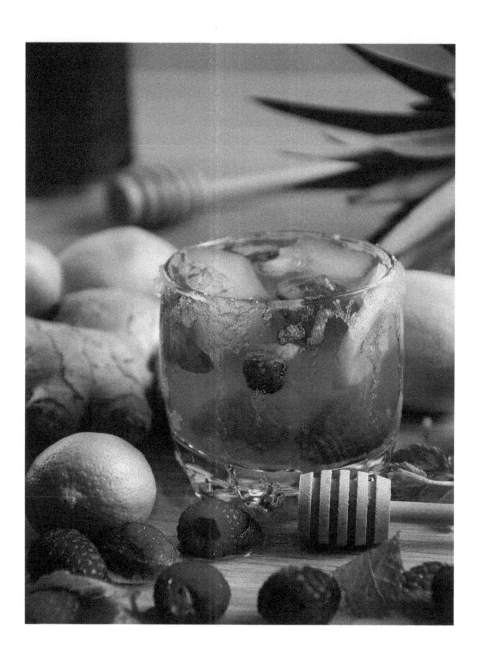

73. Mint-Citrus Iced Tea

Preparation time: 15 minutes

Cooking time: 0 minutes

Servings: 6

Ingredients:

- 6 tea

- 1/2 cup fresh mint leaves

- 3 oranges, sliced

- 3 lemons, sliced

- 3 limes, sliced

- 6 cups boiling water

- 1/4 cup granulated sugar

- 1 handful of ice cubes

Directions:

1. In a teapot, mix mint leaves, tea bags, lime, lemon, and orange slices; add boiling water and steep for at least 10

minutes. Strain it into a pitcher and stir in sugar. Serve over ice.

Nutrition:

Calories: 0

Carbs: 0g

Fat: 0g

Protein: 0g

74. Cucumber, Lemon Kiwi Agua Fresca

Preparation time: 15 minutes

Cooking time: 0 minutes

Servings: 8

Ingredients:

- 1 large cucumber, peeled and seeded

- 6 kiwis, peeled

- ½ cup lemon juice

- 2 tbsp. honey

- 6 cups water, divided

- More kiwi slices for garnish

Directions:

1. Combine cucumber, kiwi, lemon juice, honey, and 1 cup water in a blender; blend until very smooth. Pour into a serving pitcher, then mix in the remaining water. Stir in ice cubes and serve garnished with kiwi slices.

Nutrition:

Calories: 27

Carbs: 6g

Fat: 0g

Protein: 0g

75. Mint, Cucumber, Lime, and Strawberry Infused Water

Preparation time: 15 minutes

Cooking time: 0 minutes

Servings: 1

Ingredients:

- 2 limes, sliced

- ¼ cup fresh mint leaves

- 1 cup sliced cucumbers

- 1 cup sliced strawberries

- Water

- Ice cubes

Directions:

1. In a ½-gallon jar, layer lime slices, cucumbers, strawberries, and mint leaves; fill with water and stir in ice cubes. Chill for at least 10 minutes, and then enjoy!

Nutrition:

Calories: 50

Carbs: 13g

Fat: 0g Protein:0g

76. Apple Tea

Preparation time: 15 minutes

Cooking time: 0 minutes

Servings: 1

Ingredients:

- Apple juice of 1 apple

- ½ cup matcha green tea

- ¼ cup carbonated mineral water

- dash of nutmeg

- dash of cinnamon

- 1 teaspoon vanilla crème stevia

Directions:

1. Mix all the ingredients until well combined. Serve.

Nutrition:

Calories: 160

Carbs: 40g Fat: 1g .Protein: 1g

Chapter 5. Desserts

77. Baked Pomegranate Cheesecake

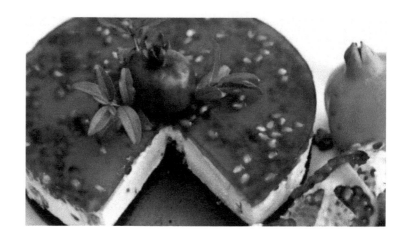

Preparation time: 15 minutes

Cooking time: 1 hour & 30 minutes

Servings: 12

Ingredients:

For the crust:

- 200 g pistachios

- 50 g powdered sugar

- ½ teaspoon ground cardamom

- 50 g melted butter

For the filling:

- 500 g cream cheese

- 200 g powdered sugar

- 30 g milk powder

- 30 grams of flour

- 300 ml sour cream

- 2 eggs, separated

- 2 tsp vanilla bean paste

- 3 sheets of gelatin

- 125 ml of water

For covering:

- 250 ml pomegranate juice

- 1 tbsp powdered sugar

- 4 sheets of gelatin

- 150 g pomegranate seeds

Directions:

1. Warm oven to 170 ° C. Line a large, loose-bottomed, straight-sided cake pan on the bottom with a piece of baking paper. Finely chop the pistachios, sugar, and cardamom with a food processor.

2. Pour in the melted butter and combine them into a paste. Press into the bottom of the prepared pan and bake for 8 minutes. Set aside to cool.

3. In a blender or by hand, stir the cream cheese and powdered sugar until creamy. Add milk powder and flour and mix well.

4. Add sour cream, egg yolks, and vanilla. Dissolve the gelatin in the water according to the package's instructions and then add to the cheesecake filling while stirring well.

5. Beat the egg whites until light and fluffy in a clean bowl. Carefully fold into the filling mixture. Rub the sides of the cooled cake pan with some butter, then add the cheesecake filling.

6. Put the pan on a large sheet of foil and crumple the foil around the sides of the can. Take a roasting tray and fill it with 5 cm of hot water.

7. Place the cheesecake in the tray and bake it in the oven for about 1 hour, still at 170 ° C. Turn off the oven and let it cool in the oven for an additional hour before allowing it to cool completely at room temperature.

8. Heat the pomegranate juice until it is warm but not bubbly. Stir in the sugar until it has dissolved. Assemble the gelatin according to the instructions in the package and add to the pomegranate juice. Let cool down to room temperature.

9. Pour about a third of the pomegranate over the cheesecake and refrigerate for 10 minutes. Repeat with the next third of the juice and refrigerate for another 10 minutes.

10. Finally, pour the last third of the juice over it, smooth it out with the back of a spoon, and spread the pomegranate seeds over it. Cover and refrigerate again for 4 hours.

Nutrition:

Calories: 380

Carbs: 42g

Fat: 22g

78. Meringues with Black Currants

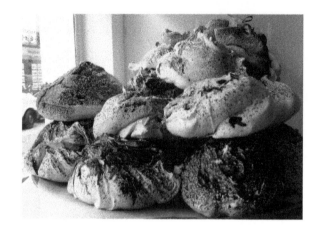

Preparation time: 15 minutes

Cooking time: 1 hour & 40 minutes

Servings: 6

Ingredients:

- 250 g black currants, washed and stems removed

- 1 heaping tablespoon of powdered sugar

- 3 large egg whites

- 100 g powdered sugar

- 150 ml double cream

Directions:

1. Warm oven to 130 ° C. Line a baking sheet with parchment paper or a silicone sheet. Put the black currants in a pan with a little cold water. Bring to a boil and simmer gently within 10 minutes.

2. Press through a sieve, then add the powdered sugar while it is still warm and stir to dissolve. Let cool down. Put the egg whites in a clean bowl and beat with an electric whisk until stiff peaks form.

3. Keep beating as the sugar is added gradually. Continue beating until the meringue is thick and shiny, then stir in about 2 tablespoons of the fruit puree, but don't stir in thoroughly.

4. Place the meringue on the prepared tray to get 12 equal blobs. Bake for 1½ hours, then remove from the oven and let cool down completely.

5. Whip the cream lightly and pour the meringues on top in pairs. Serve with the remaining black currant sauce.

Nutrition:

Calories: 121

Carbs: 26g

Fat: 0g Protein: 2g

79. Black Currant and Raspberry Granita

Preparation time: 15 minutes

Cooking time: 0 minutes

Servings: 2

Ingredients:

- 150 g black currants, washed and stems removed

- 150 g raspberries

- 50 g powdered sugar

Directions:

1. Beat the black currants and raspberries in a blender or food processor. Pass through a sieve to the skins.

2. Fold the powdered sugar into the fruit puree and stir to dissolve. Transfer to an airtight container and freeze within 2 hours.

3. Take it out of the freezer and let it sit at room temperature for 10 to 15 minutes (or use the defrost

setting in the microwave for about 30 seconds). Crush the mixture into crystals with a fork and serve immediately.

Nutrition:

Calories: 50

Carbs: 12g

Fat: 0g

Protein: 0g

80. Chocolate and Blackberry Mini Pavlovas

Preparation time: 15 minutes

Cooking time: 45 minutes

Servings: 8

Ingredients:

- 6 large egg whites

- 200 g powdered sugar

- 50 g cocoa powder

- 1 teaspoon balsamic vinegar

- 50 g high quality (70%) dark chocolate, chopped

For covering:

- 300 ml double cream

- 100 g powdered sugar

- 500 g blackberries

- 30 g of good (70%) dark chocolate, grated

Directions:

1. Warm oven to 190 ° C. Line a large baking sheet with parchment paper or a silicone sheet. Put the egg whites in your large bowl, then whisk until stiff peaks form.

2. Stir in the sugar a tablespoon at a time and keep stirring until stiff and shiny. Add the cocoa, balsamic vinegar, and chocolate. Fold until everything is well mixed.

3. Scoop the meringue into eight roughly even servings on the baking sheet and flatten the top of each. Put in the oven, then reduce the oven temperature immediately to 160 ° C and cook for about 45 minutes.

4. When cooked, the meringues should be firm and crispy on the sides and top but still a little squidgy on the inside. Turn off the oven, open the door a little and let it slowly cool in the oven for another half an hour.

5. Remove the meringues on individual serving plates. Whisk the cream until it keeps its shape. Add powdered sugar and whisk again.

6. Stack the cream on top of each meringue and spread the blackberries on top. Sprinkle over the grated chocolate.

Nutrition:

Calories: 115

Carbs: 27g

Fat: 0g /Protein: 0g

81. Chocolate Mousse

Preparation time: 15 minutes

Cooking time: 0 minutes

Servings: 8

Ingredients:

- 170 g of good quality dark chocolate (70%), broken into small pieces

- 20 g butter

- 4 large eggs, separated

Directions:

1. Place a small heat-resistant bowl over a pan of lightly boiling water, making sure that the bowl's bottom does not touch the water.

2. Place the chocolate and butter in the bowl and slowly heat them until they are almost melted. Remove from heat and stir until thick and shiny.

3. Beat the egg yolks lightly and pour them into the melted chocolate one by one. Stir continuously until the yolk is completely incorporated. Place the egg whites in a clean bowl and use an electric whisk to whisk the egg whites until stiff peaks form.

4. Put a third of the egg white to the melted chocolate and mix well. Then very carefully fold in the rest of the egg white, trying not to knock the air out of the egg white. Spread the mousse over four casserole dishes and chill for 1–2 hours before serving.

Nutrition:

Calories: 94

Carbs: 13g

Fat: 3g

Protein: 3g

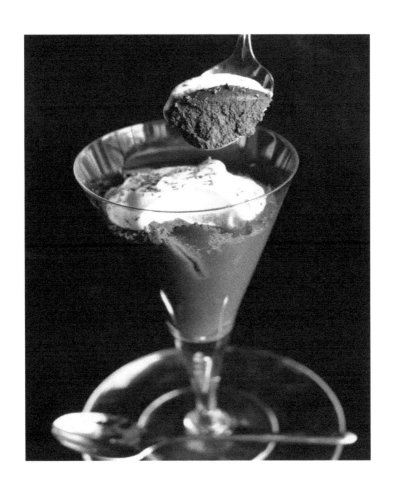

82. Green Iced Tea Ice-cream

Preparation time: 15 minutes

Cooking time: 0 minutes

Servings: 6

Ingredients:

- 600 ml of skimmed milk

- 150 g powdered sugar a pinch of salt

- 30 g matcha green tea powder

Directions:

1. Put milk, sugar, and salt in a saucepan. Heat on medium heat until it only steams; after that, stir in the green tea powder.

2. Continue whisking until mixture begins to foam and steam, but remove from heat before it begins to boil. Cool the mixture in the pan, transfer it to a bowl or jug, cover and refrigerate for 1–2 hours.

3. When completely cool, place in a pre-chilled ice maker and stir for 20 to 30 minutes, then transfer to an airtight container and freeze.

4. Remove from the freezer 5 minutes before serving. Spread over four casserole dishes or small dishes and chill for 1–2 hours before serving.

Nutrition:

Calories: 120

Carbs: 17g

Fat: 5g- protein 2g

83. Pomegranate and Blueberry Rice

Preparation time: 15 minutes

Cooking time: 0 minutes

Servings: 2

Ingredients:

- 1 teaspoon matcha green tea powder

- 100 g blueberries (fresh or frozen)

- 100 ml pomegranate juice

- 150 g ice cubes

Directions:

1. Stir the matcha powder in half a cup of hot water until it has dissolved. Set aside to cool. Puree the blueberries with a food processor or blender. Add pomegranate juice, matcha tea, and ice cubes and stir until smooth. Serve immediately.

Nutrition:

Calories: 52

Carbs: 13g Fat: 1g .Protein: 1g

84. Chocolate Apple Cake

Preparation time: 15 minutes

Cooking time: 30 minutes

Servings: 4

Ingredients:

- 4 apples, peeled, pitted, and cut into small pieces

- Juice of ½ lemon

- 20 g soft light brown sugar

- 1 tbsp brandy

- 50 ml of water

- 50 g powdered sugar

- 1 tbsp cocoa powder

- 30 g ground almonds

- 1 large egg white

Directions:

1. Preheat the oven to 160 ° C. Put the chopped apple in a saucepan with lemon juice, brown sugar, brandy, and water.

2. Boil, adjust the heat, and cook covered for 5 minutes. Uncover, turn up the heat and cook for another 5 minutes until the sauce has thickened.

3. Mix the powdered sugar, cocoa, and ground almonds in a bowl. In a clean bowl, whisk the egg white until it forms stiff peaks, then fold into the dry ingredients.

4. Divide the cooked apple into four individual serving dishes or casserole dishes. Spoon the topping over the apple and gently shake or tap it to smooth the mixture. Place the casserole dishes on a baking sheet and bake for 20 minutes.

Nutrition:

Calories: 330

Carbs: 44g

Fat: 15g

Protein: 3g

85. Blueberry Fun

Preparation time: 15 minutes

Cooking time: 0 minutes

Servings: 4

Ingredients:

- 500 g blueberries

- 400 g natural yogurt

- 50 ml crème fraîche

- 2 lemon peel

- ½ teaspoon ground cinnamon

- 30 g powdered sugar

Directions:

1. Set aside a handful of blueberries. Put the remaining blueberries in a food processor or blender and stir until smooth. If you want, you can strain the blueberries through a sieve at this point to remove the peel.

2. Mix the yogurt, crème fraîche, lemon zest, ground cinnamon, and powdered sugar in a bowl. Fold in the blueberry sauce very carefully.

3. Divide the fool into four serving glasses or casserole dishes and place the reserved blueberries on top. Chill for within 30 minutes before serving.

Nutrition:

Calories: 100

Carbs: 13g

Fat: 5g

Protein: 1g

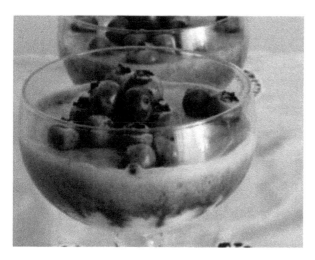

86. Berry Good!

Preparation time: 15 minutes

Cooking time: 10 minutes

Servings: 8

Ingredients:

- 250 g strawberries, peeled and roughly chopped

- 250 g raspberries

- 250 g black currants, washed and stems removed

- 50 g powdered sugar

- 100 ml of water

- 50 ml sherry

- 200 g sponge cake

- 200 ml double cream

- 200 g pudding

Directions:

1. Put the strawberries, raspberries, and black currants in a saucepan with the sugar and 100 ml of water.

2. Bring to a boil and simmer for 10 minutes. Remove from heat and stir in sherry. Separate the juice from the berries by pouring it through a sieve and saving both.

3. Pour the juice into the large glass bowl. Cut the sponge cake into small pieces and the cake into the juice at the bottom of the bowl to form a generous layer. Place half of the berries on top.

Nutrition:

Calories: 280

Carbs: 70g

Fat: 1g

Protein: 14g

87. Snowflakes

Preparation time: 15 minutes

Cooking time: 10 minutes

Servings: 1

Ingredients:

- Won ton wrappers

- Oil to frying

- Powdered sugar

Directions:

1. Cut won ton wrappers just like you'd a snowflake. Heat oil. When hot, add wonton, fry for approximately 30 seconds, then flip over. Drain on a paper towel, then shower with powdered sugar.

Nutrition:

Calories: 96

Carbs: 24.1g

Fat: 0.6g Protein: 2.8g

88. Home-Made Marshmallow Fluff

Preparation time: 15 minutes

Cooking time: 20 minutes

Servings: 4

Ingredients:

- 3/4 cup sugar

- 1/2 cup light corn syrup

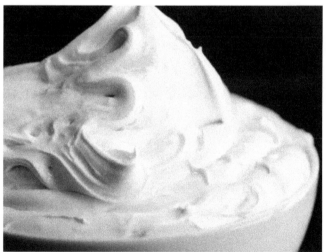

- 1/4 cup water

- 1/8 teaspoon salt

- 3 little egg whites

- 1/4 teaspoon cream of tartar

- 1 teaspoon 1/2 teaspoon vanilla extract

Directions:

1. In a small pan, mix sugar, corn syrup, salt, and water. Put a candy thermometer to the side of this pan, but make sure it will not touch the pan's underside.

2. From the bowl of a stand mixer, combine egg whites and cream of tartar. Begin to whip on medium speed with the whisk attachment.

3. Meanwhile, turn a burner on top and place the pan with the sugar mix onto heat. Pout mix into a boil and heat to 240 degrees, stirring periodically.

4. The aim is to have the egg whites whipped to soft peaks and also the sugar heated to 240 degrees at near the same moment. Simply stop stirring the egg whites once they hit soft peaks.

5. Once the sugar has already reached 240 amounts, turn heat low allowing it to reduce. Insert a little quantity of the sugar mix and let it mix. Put another bit of the sugar mix. Add mixture slowly, and that means you never scramble the egg whites.

6. After all of the sugar was added to the egg whites, then decrease the mixer's speed and keep mixing the concoction for around 7- 9 minutes until the fluff remains glossy and stiff.

7. At roughly the 5-minute mark, then add the vanilla extract. Use fluff immediately or store in an airtight container in the fridge for around two weeks.

Nutrition:

Calories: 23

Carbs: 5.8g

Protein: 0.1g

Fat: 0g

89. Banana Ice Cream

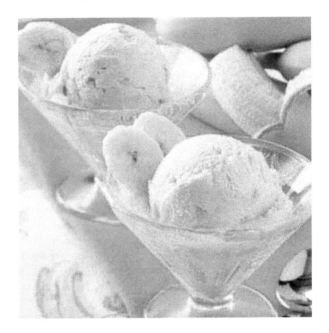

Preparation time: 15 minutes

Cooking time: 0 minutes

Servings: 3

Ingredients:

- 3 quite ripe banana - peeled and chopped

- A couple of chocolate chips

- 2 tbsp skim milk

Directions:

1. Throw all fixing into a food processor and blend until creamy. Freeze and appreciate afterward.

Nutrition:

Calories: 387

Carbs: 47.3g

Fat: 19.5g –Protein 6.3g

90. Dark Chocolate Pretzel Cookies

Preparation time: 15 minutes

Cooking time: 20 minutes

Servings: 4

Ingredients:

- 1 cup yogurt

- 1/2 teaspoon baking soda

- 1/4 teaspoon salt

- 1/4 teaspoon cinnamon

- 4 butter (softened/0

- 1/3 cup brown sugar

- 1 egg

- 1/2 teaspoon vanilla

- 1/2 cup dark chocolate chips

- 1/2 cup pretzels, chopped

Directions:

1. Preheat oven to 350 degrees. Mix the sugar, butter, vanilla, and egg in a medium bowl. Mix the flour, baking soda, plus salt in another bowl.

2. Stir the bread mixture in, using all the wet components, along with the chocolate chips and pretzels until just blended. Drop a large spoonful of dough on an unlined baking sheet.

3. Bake within 15-17 minutes, or until the bottoms are somewhat all crispy. Allow cooling on a wire rack.

Nutrition:

Calories: 300

Carbs: 44.3g

Fat: 11.2g

Protein: 3.8g

Conclusion

Congratulations! You now know how to follow the Sirtfood diet diligently and lose weight healthily and consistently.

There are several diets out there. Dieting has become an industry of its own, with videos, books, blogs, and all sorts of diet pills, supplements, and other items accessible to customers. At the same time, Western nations are becoming more health-conscious and overweight, and, as a result, there is a rising demand for information on diets and items related to weight loss. However, what's not much of it is solid, useful information about how to successfully diet-that is, how to effectively lose weight and keep it off.

Anyone can lose weight by following one of the many fad diets available. Still, these diets have a few fatal flaws. They generally do not provide you with a nutritionally healthy diet; they're not intended for anything other than short-term weight loss and, perhaps worst of all, they generally do not provide you with any sleep.

However, you don't need fad diet plans or diet pills to eat effectively; you need the right details on what to do and what to avoid when you're trying to lose weight. The SirtFood diet is 70-80 percent raw and also contains the following:

Motivation: If you are not motivated to lose weight and improve your health, you probably won't be successful regardless of what kind of diet you follow. It needs the self-discipline to avoid food mistakes, and to get enough exercise, you need to lose weight and keep it off. Without that, nothing is going to work for you in the long run.

Water: Drinking plenty of water is something you can do in the first place because it is so crucial to good health. Drinking eight or more cups of water a day helps your digestive system work more efficiently, helping you lose weight, and drinking water also helps you feel full; in many cases, you may be thirsty when you feel hungry. Drink a glass of water when you're feeling hungry and make a point of getting a glass before meals; you might be shocked by how much less you consume by mealtimes.

Daily Drill: We all know that we need regular exercise, especially if we're trying to lose weight. If you're not getting some form of exercise regularly, try starting small with a half-hour walk every day and work your way up to more intensive exercise and longer workouts. Usually, you'll get the best results with half an hour to 45 minutes of exercise at least three or four days a week. Even if you don't have a lot of spare time on your day, try to put in a little physical exercise whenever you can, take the stairs instead of the elevator, walk to the store instead of driving, or to take a cab, and so on – every little bit helps you lose excess weight and keep it off.

Good, Nutritionally Balanced Diets: We all have an excellent idea of what we should eat; fresh vegetables and fruit, whole grains, small amounts of healthy fats like olive oil, fish, and other lean meats. It is more important to keep your mind clear: refined flours, sugar, processed foods, and any food or beverage filled with preservatives and other artificial ingredients. Get into the habit of carefully reading food labels and, if possible, cook your food with fresh ingredients instead of purchasing pre-made packaged food. It's OK to get a little out of your diet once in a while. But most of the time, you need to stick to the plan.

When you get used to eating healthy, you will find that you quickly lose your appetite for less nutritious choices, and, combined with daily exercise, it will make it easier to stay away from the weight you've gained.

Lightning Source UK Ltd.
Milton Keynes UK
UKHW020234220521
384136UK00001B/6